AGILE IMPLEMENTATION

AGILE
IMPLEMENTATION

*A Model for Implementing Evidence-Based
Healthcare Solutions into Real-World Practice
to Achieve Sustainable Change*

MALAZ BOUSTANI, MD, MPH
JOSE AZAR, MD
CRAIG A. SOLID, PHD

NEW YORK

LONDON • NASHVILLE • MELBOURNE • VANCOUVER

AGILE IMPLEMENTATION

A Model for Implementing Evidence-Based
Healthcare Solutions into Real-World Practice
to Achieve Sustainable Change

© 2020 **MALAZ BOUSTANI**, MD, MPH , **JOSE AZAR**, MD ,
CRAIG A. SOLID, PHD

Published in New York, New York, by Morgan James Publishing. Morgan James is a trademark of Morgan James, LLC. www.MorganJamesPublishing.com

ISBN 978-1-64279-659-9 eBook
ISBN 978-1-64279-658-2 hardcover
Library of Congress Control Number: 2019907494

Cover Design by:
Rachel Lopez
www.r2cdesign.com

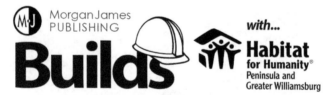

Morgan James is a proud partner of Habitat for Humanity Peninsula and Greater Williamsburg. Partners in building since 2006.

Get involved today! Visit
www.MorganJamesBuilds.com

Table of Contents

Acknowledgements

Malaz Boustani, M.D., MPH

This book is an attempt to cultivate passionate, resilient, and innovative change agents who share one vision of transforming the current healthcare system into a smart, agile, social organism capable of delivering safe, highly reliable, evidence-based, and personalized medical services for everyone, everywhere. Together, I'm hopeful that we will protect the brain and the health of millions of families including our own. I am indebted to many people who have helped me on my journey and who I would like to acknowledge, including my amazing family, friends, mentors, mentees, students, scientists, and clinicians. There are a few people who I would like to name who have had a significant impact on my development along the way. My Wife, Mary Boustani, who taught me that there is no "p-value" in the boardroom, coached me on how to develop partnerships with healthcare administrators, and helped me understand the importance of learning about the needs of my clinicians and patients. I am forever grateful for how she tolerates my long hours and frequent travels. My daughter, Katreen Boustani, the family "social informatician," has been instrumental in helping me master mindfulness, has challenged my thinking and approach, and has kept me connected to a younger generation. My son, Zayn Boustani, instilled in me a deep appreciation of the art and the value of associate thinking and deep observation to the creation of innovative solutions capable of solving problems at the personal level of each patient, each clinician, and each system. While I was at UNC, Dr. Jan Busby Whitehead was my fellowship director and was instrumental in my development as a scientist. The personalized curriculum and individual guidance allowed me to grow and develop as a researcher and has enabled me to examine situations in an objective and logical manner. I am forever grateful to Dr. Christopher Callahan for not only recruiting me to Indiana University, but for his advice and guidance regarding research, leadership, and funding, and for becoming a great friend. I want to thank Dr. Lisa Harris for giving me the opportunity and the resources to develop the Health Aging Brain Center and the Critical care Recovery center at Eskenazi Health. She took away the walls between research and clinical services and supported our efforts of creating the Office of Research and Development at Eskenazi Health. My work in implementation science would not have started at all without the vision and the support of my mentor, Dr. Anantha Shekhar. His belief in the generalizability of our work in brain care into the entire healthcare transformation process and his vision of the value of implementation science in shortening and optimizing the discovery-to-delivery translational cycle were simply second to none. Finally, I want to thank my amazing groups of mentees and students who took a risk by selecting me as their mentor and coach for the past decade. I learned a lot from this group of disruptive innovators. Thank you, Noll, Babar, Nicole, Patrick, Sophia, Eric, Archita, Nadia, Ashely, Cathy, and Michael.

Jose Azar, M.D.

I am passionate about eliminating suffering from cancer and improving the care delivered by healthcare delivery systems. I pursue these goals by leading the development of agile learning organizations and by leading diverse and inter-professional teams that can rapidly and effectively implement innovative solutions to healthcare. From an initial interest in quality and patient safety, I have been a student, then an educator, a leader, an innovator, and a developer of the novel method of Agile Implementation. By helping to co-found the Center and the Certificate for Health Innovation and Implementation Science, I hope to disseminate this method and develop a network of passionate and resilient change agents who are capable of transforming healthcare to a safe, high quality, equitable, affordable and personalized service.

I am grateful for all the experiences and opportunities I have been given along this journey.

I am most grateful for Karen, my soulmate (Rouheh), for teaching me to be "real" and true to myself. For believing in me and for being the wind under my wings. For all the wisdom and fun we have exchanged. For teaching me by example how to be a servant leader. For picking me up every time I fall, for inspiring me to dream big, for helping me believe that everything is possible. Thank you for always bringing out the best in me.

I am grateful for my children, Christopher and Nicole. You are my joy and you continuously help me become the best version of myself. Our debates have always challenged and refined my thinking. Your pursuit of excellence and your resilience in martial arts and ballet have inspired me and motivated me. You have taught me to learn and grow from failure. I admire you and look forward to seeing you making this world a better place for all.

I am grateful for my parents, for raising me through the adversity of life in Lebanon during a civil war and for always believing that I can be the best. I'm grateful for my sister Lynn, for always keeping me humble, challenging me to achieve more and for being there for me every time I fell down.

I am grateful for my Level Ten Martial Arts School, Master Theros and Associate Master Tucher, for teaching me and helping me develop resilience and discipline.

I am grateful for Dr. Ryan Nagy for our friendship, for giving me the chance to do what I love and for mentoring me on leading a complex organization through change and tough times. For Drs. Jeffrey Rothenberg and Michael Niemeyer, for identifying my talent and believing in me. Dr. Jonathan Gottlieb for mentoring me and challenging me. Dr. Michele Saysana for the friendship and all the support.

I am grateful for Jennifer Dunscomb and Kristen Kelley for inspiring me, for challenging me and for teaching me how to listen and effectively lead change in the real world. I am also grateful to all the clinical nurse specialists, the quality improvement consultants, infection preventionists, nurses, physicians and healthcare professional teams at IU Health for making a difference in patients' lives every day.

I am grateful for all my mentees and students for always inspiring me and challenging me to be the best version of myself. I have learned so much from all of you.

I am grateful for Dr. Larry Cripe, my teacher and my dear friend, for always challenging me to aspire for more, to think more analytically, and for being my moral compass. I will always cherish our monthly reflections.

Finally, and most importantly, I am very grateful for Dr. Malaz Boustani, my mentor and my dear friend, for choosing me as his experiment and for all the dedication to my mentorship. Thank you for teaching me to never be complacent, and to always dream big! Thank you for challenging me to accomplish more when I succeeded, and for lifting me up when I failed. Thank you for all the tough, judgement-free, and honest feedback that has helped me refine and sharpen myself. I would have never accomplished what I have without you.

Craig A. Solid, PhD

I first and foremost want to thank my co-authors for sharing their personal and professional experiences with me, which are reflected in the stories contained in this book. I see them as not just illustrations of the effectiveness of the Agile Implementation model, but as formative, impactful, and sometimes difficult experiences that healthcare professionals face on a daily basis. I am proud to be part of the collaboration that helped bring those stories to life. I would like to say a special thank you to Dr. Boustani for his guidance and council over the past two years and over multiple collaborations. His energy and optimism are infectious, and I have truly enjoyed working with him. I of course cannot say enough about the love and support I have received from my family, without whom none of what I do would matter. Thank you.

Introduction
By Dr. Malaz Boustani

I have been practicing medicine, conducting clinical research, and mentoring scientists for more than two decades. Without exception, the doctors, nurses, social workers, and healthcare administrators I have encountered on my journey are passionately committed to providing the best possible care to patients and their families.

In pursuit of fulfilling this commitment, most providers invest significant time and effort to stay current on the latest and most effective medical discoveries, including devices, drugs, and models of care. These passionate and resilient healthcare providers try various strategies to incorporate these new methods and ideas into daily practice. Unfortunately, in doing so they battle a mountain of constraints, including limited time, tight budgets, and ever-increasing oversight and governance. Integrating novel methods or practices identified in clinical research into real-world practice is a struggle against routines, limited resources, and the very real issue of provider burnout.

Some estimates put the average time for proven clinical research to reach clinical practice at 17 years.[1,2] When I first read this figure, I was staggered. Considering that these innovations occur multiple times a year, I found the prospect of these revolutionary discoveries collecting dust on the shelf unthinkable. No one would argue that 17 years is a reasonable length of time to implement care practices demonstrated to be effective. However, even when evidence-based services are implemented, there is no guarantee they will be sustained, adapted, or distributed across the healthcare delivery organization. Conversely, I have seen ineffective or even harmful practices remain in operation after evidence revealed that they should be discontinued. As a result, the majority of patients today receive healthcare services unsupported by a high level of evidence.[3] In fact, significant numbers of patients experience harm and even deaths that may be preventable.[4]

Today's Healthcare System
Healthcare 1.0

I have always considered myself as much a scientist as a physician. Early in my training, I was exposed to how prevalent chronic diseases like osteoarthritis, Alzheimer's disease, depression, diabetes, coronary artery disease, and heart failure were among older people. I quickly realized—as a scientist—that if I lived as long as I hoped to, there was a good chance I would have to deal with one or more of these chronic diseases. Of all the chronic diseases, those affecting the brain scared me the most, and I became increasingly aware of the challenges these patients (and their families) faced.

With that heightened focus during my medical residency, I began to take notice of shortcomings within the current healthcare delivery system (healthcare 1.0), even with its

1 IN 4 😕😐😕💀 HARMED

$750B WASTED SPENDING

50% 😐✗ RECEIVE NO EVIDENCE BASED CARE

75,000 DEATHS💀

30% WASTED ANNUAL SPENDING

Sources: 74K death, and 30% wasted annual cite Smith M, Saunders R, Stuckhardt L, McGinnis JM. Best care at lower cost: the path to continuously learning health care in America:. National Academies Press; 2013. Institute of Medicine. 2013. Best Care at Lower Cost: The Path to Continuously Learning Health Care in America. Washington, DC: The National Academies Press. https://doi.org/10.17226/13444.

The 1 in 4 experience harms cite Landrigan C, Parry G, Bones C, Hackbarth A, Goldmann D, Sharek P. Temporal Trends in Rates of Patient Harm Resulting from Medical Care. The New England Journal of Medicine 2010 Nov;363:2124—34. Ebell MH, Sokol R, Lee A, Simons C, Early J. How good is the evidence to support primary care practice? Evid Based Med 2017;22:88–92.

50% do not receive evidence based is Ebell MH, Sokol R, Lee A, Simons C, Early J. How good is the evidence to support primary care practice? Evid Based Med. 2017;22:88–92.

highly educated, dedicated, and caring workforce serving the personalized and complex needs of patients and families living with Alzheimer's disease. Healthcare professionals did not have the tools, time, or resources to provide the necessary care and support to these patients and their loved ones. I witnessed

THE CURRENT STATE OF AGING BRAIN CARE IN THE US

AS MANY AS

82%

OF THOSE WITH COGNITIVE IMPAIRMENT HAVE BEHAVIORAL SYMPTOMS

AS MANY AS

20% OF

FDA-APPROVED MEDICATIONS CAN HAVE ADVERSE COGNITIVE EFFECTS

UP TO

80%

OF DEMENTIA CASES ARE UNRECOGNIZED

APPROXIMATELY ONE-FOURTH

ARE PRESCRIBED MEDICATIONS THAT CAN HAVE ADVERSE COGNITIVE EFFECT

UP TO 25%

ARE PRESCRIBED "OFF LABEL PSYCHOTROPICS" USE

49% OF PATIENTS **AND 21%** OF CAREGIVERS VISIT THE ER EACH YEAR

26% OF PATIENTS **AND 11%** OF CAREGIVERS HAVE A HOSPITAL VISIT EACH YEAR

THE AVERAGE LENGTH OF STAY IN THE HOSPITAL MAY BE UP TO **9.2 DAYS**

Sources: LaMantia et al, ADAD 2016; French et al, Health Affairs 2014; Khan et al JHM 2012; Boustani et al, JGIM 2012; Boustani et al, Aging and Mental Health 2011; Boustani et al, JHM 2010; Schubert et al, JGIM 2008; Schubert et al, JAGS 2006; Callahan et al, JAMA 2006; Boustani et al, JGIM 2005; Boustani et al, Ann Int Med 2003

numerous families wilt under the burden of caring for someone experiencing declining cognition. This revelation was a turning point for me. Understanding and improving brain health became my passion and my calling.

After my time as a resident, I went to the University of North Carolina (Chapel Hill) for a fellowship to learn how to be a scientist. My hope was to discover ways to provide better protection for the brain—the only organ, I noted, that you cannot transplant or replace. My time at UNC was extraordinary. I was fortunate to have an excellent fellowship director who saw that I was driven and passionate about brain health, and who personalized the curriculum and offered me individual guidance. This fellowship equipped me with priceless competencies and tools that allowed me to detect relevant signals among reams of data; identify gaps in the scientific literature; design innovative models of brain care; secure funding to conduct rigorous research studies to evaluate the efficacy of these innovative models; and share my results with the world via national presentations and peer-reviewed papers. At UNC I became a physician scientist on a mission to transform brain health.

In the summer of 2002, after my geriatric clinical research fellowship, I was fortunate to be recruited by Dr. Christopher Callahan to come to Indiana University as assistant professor of medicine and scientist at his Center for Aging Research within the Regenstrief Institute. Chris agreed to be my mentor; he also became my friend and later stood up as the best man in my wedding. He spent countless hours coaching me on how to lead a research team, how to build a clinical laboratory, how to secure federal research funding, how to use storytelling to share my research findings, and how to use health information technology to support healthcare providers at the point of care where they make their crucial clinical decisions.

With support from the federal government, our IU team designed a new care model for Alzheimer's disease and completed a randomized controlled trial (the gold standard study design to

find out if a treatment actually works) to evaluate the efficacy of our care model. The data from the trial found that our model worked: it reduced the behavioral and psychological disabilities of Alzheimer's disease, including wandering, agitation, and depression. Furthermore, our model decreased the stress of the unpaid caregivers supporting the patients living with this devastating brain disease. Notably, the model provided the necessary help without increasing prescriptions for potential harmful psychotropic medications for patients.

With such positive results, in 2006 Chris and I began sharing our results with the scientific community across the globe. At the same time as our research success, the geriatric clinic within the hospital where I worked had to make cuts, and despite the fact that I had just received a prestigious research career development award (I was named a Paul Beeson Aging Research Scholar), I lost my clinical geriatric position. Knowing my passion for brain health, the leadership at Eskenazi Health in Indianapolis reached out shortly afterward to offer me a position within their urban health system where I conducted most of my clinical research studies. Although grateful and excited for the opportunity to continue my work as a geriatrician, I made it clear to them that if I accepted, I wanted to build a center for brain health. They agreed with only one condition: the entire center had to be ready within four months.

With new direction and a tight deadline looming, I immersed myself in complexity theory and other frameworks to tackle this huge undertaking. Understanding how health systems function would allow me to identify and dissect the factors associated with practice and process adoption by providers. I had earned an opportunity to make a positive impact in my fight against Alzheimer's disease, but for it to succeed I needed to ensure the sustainability of the new brain center. My previous experiences with change models like Lean and Plan-Do-Study-Act (PDSA) left me wanting more. They felt incomplete in their approach to affecting change to the care delivery system given the complexities inherent in the daily activities and interactions of the individuals operating therein. There was also the issue of the inconsistency in their effectiveness: why did PDSA work sometimes and not others? Was it a matter of execution, or was it simply beyond the model's capabilities to provide the necessary results in some circumstances or settings? When it did work, what was driving the change, and was that a characteristic of the implementation method or something else?

IMPLEMENTATION SCIENCE

DEVELOPING TOOLS, PROCESSES, AND STRATEGIES FOR RAPID, EFFICIENT, SCALABLE, AND SUSTAINABLE IMPLEMENTATION OF EVIDENCE-BASED SERVICES IN THE LOCAL "REAL WORLD"

I have always been a curious person who sought to understand *why* something happens and *how* things work. That drive for answers led me on my path as both a physician and a scientist, dedicated to implementing long-lasting and evidence-supported planned change. Motivated by the need to create and build the center for brain health, I began to see how different theoretical frameworks of complex systems and human behavior fit together to accurately describe how care delivery systems (and their members) functioned and interacted. These insights have allowed my colleagues and me to develop our own model for implementing evidence-based solutions in real-world situations with a high level of success and sustainability. We call it Agile Implementation.

In the chapters that follow, we will walk through specific examples that illustrate and demonstrate how the Agile Implementation model addresses the unique nature of care delivery systems. Together we will follow the narrative of the problem and the steps we took to arrive at a process for implementing evidence-based care solutions. Afterwards, we will explore in detail the underlying theories and frameworks upon which our model is built. Finally, we will describe the steps of the model and explain how they leverage the lessons learned from our experiences and theories of complexity and behavioral economics.

I am excited to take you on this journey. When I started exploring these concepts my aim was to create a system all providers could use to improve healthcare. After years of dedicated work, I am proud to present you with the path I walked to arrive at Agile Implementation. From theory to experiment to sustainable model, I thank you for the opportunity to present my research. As you will see, Agile Implementation has been a solution for creating sustainable and efficient change in how to care for patients (and their unpaid caregivers) living with

Alzheimer's disease, and those who survived a crucial illness and a stay in the intensive care units. I am excited to show you how it can transform your health environments as well.

Part I

CASE STUDIES

Chapter 1

The Story of the Healthy Aging Brain Center

Alzheimer's disease is a complex brain disease. It takes away the cognitive ability of millions of people to function independently in their own homes and communities. The most common form of dementia, it affects one out of 10 to one out of three older adults. For these individuals, completing a simple task such as dressing, eating, or walking becomes a major battle. This devastating disease robs them of the ability to manage their own health by limiting their capability to reach out to their physicians, follow medical instructions (such as taking the right medications at the right time for the right dose), and navigate the complex healthcare system or related financial systems.

A large proportion of people living with Alzheimer's disease become victims of car accidents, financial exploitation, or a variety of injuries. Furthermore, these vulnerable individuals suffer from depression, anxiety, insomnia, and false beliefs. The cluster of cognitive, physical, and psychological disabilities of this disease and the enormous burden on the family members caring for those living with Alzheimer's disease imperil the ability of our current healthcare system tremendously. Both patients and their families are frequently in and out of hospitals and emergency departments and often endure medical complications and adverse effects. This terrible disease not only takes away the independence of these five million patients, but it imposes a significant emotional, financial, and physical burden on the millions of families and friends who often provide the first line—and sometimes the only line—of support and care. These unpaid caregivers may spend hundreds of hours each month providing care[5] and trying to navigate our country's complex health care system. The pressure of caring for patients living with Alzheimer's can be so enormous that these unpaid caregivers may experience high levels of stress, and often their own health, quality of life, finances, and independence deteriorates.[6,7]

In a nutshell, for each Alzheimer's diagnosis there are in fact *two* individuals living with the disease that the healthcare system must care for: the person whose brain cells are dying from the toxic protein called amyloid and the unpaid caregiver.

$5.7 MILLION INDIVIDUALS w/ALZHEIMER'S

YEARLY COST OF DEMENTIA PER INDIVIDUAL
$56,290

18.4B
HOURS OF CARE PROVIDED

78% PERCENT OF TIME SPENT IS BY INFORMAL CARE GIVERS

Sources: Alzheimer's Association Facts and Figures (2018): https://www.alz.org/media/ HomeOffice/Facts%20and%20Figures/facts-and-figures.pdf; Hurd MD, Martorell P, Delavande A, Mullen KJ, Langa KM. Monetary costs of dementia in the United States. N Engl J Med. Apr 04 2013;368(14):1326-1334.; Friedman EM, Shih RA, Langa KM, Hurd MD. US Prevalence And Predictors Of Informal Caregiving For Dementia. Health Aff (Millwood). Oct 2015;34(10):1637-1641.

The Burden of Alzheimer's Disease

Most physicians realized many years ago that the care delivery system was not designed to provide proper care for patients living with Alzheimer's disease and their unpaid caregivers. It is simply not possible to adequately address the unique needs of those living with Alzheimer's in a single setting or over the course of disjointed and unrelated office visits. If we were going to provide the appropriate care—care that was individualized, ongoing, and effective regardless of the setting—it was necessary to develop a new system that reinvented and reimagined how these patients were cared for and also addressed the needs of the unpaid caregivers.

In 2007, almost all patients living with Alzheimer's disease cared for at Eskenazi Health were done so by primary care clinicians with no additional support. No care or structured support was provided for the unpaid caregivers. Eskenazi Health is a safety-net integrated urban healthcare system serving the healthcare needs of Marion County residents in Indiana, although its care of Alzheimer's disease was typical of healthcare systems across the country, primarily because of how national billing and reimbursement systems were structured. Hospitals and doctors who saw patients billed Medicare and other insurers for tests that were ordered and medical services they performed. However, coverage was (and still is) often limited to medical services performed for the patient (not the unpaid caregiver) and for only those services that occurred during the hospital or office visit. This payment model was not aligned with the medical, psychological, and social needs of patients living with Alzheimer's disease and their unpaid caregivers.

Alzheimer's disease affects every aspect of an individual's life, but these patients were typically only receiving medical care during the short periods when they were in front of a physician. The consequences were suboptimal outcomes and excessive costs of care. To illustrate what could happen, let's consider a patient living with Alzheimer's who develops an infection in the lungs (pneumonia). For this patient, their cognitive disability delays early detection and early treatment of the infection, eventually exacerbating the infection into a severe case that requires a hospitalization. In the hospital, the patient may get very confused and agitated and may be unable to pay attention, making them vulnerable to adverse events such as falls or pulling out intravenous catheterization, as well as inhibiting their ability to cooperate with medical care. These inattentive, confused, and disoriented patients often stop eating and subsequently get weak and unsteady and suffer from multiple hospital-acquired complications such as bed sores and broken hips.

Something needed to be done. Improving care for patients living with Alzheimer's disease wasn't just something that would be welcome, it was a necessity and personal. I have lost family members to this devastating disease. Fortunately, calls for change did not fall on deaf ears, and leadership at Eskenazi Health agreed that there was a meaningful opportunity that warranted massive action and change. Specifically, providing excellent brain care was part of Eskenazi's mission to serve the health of its community. The Eskenazi leadership mantra was and still is that *"There is no Health without Brain Health."*

The year before this opportunity was identified at Eskenazi Health, the results of two randomized controlled trials on a new Alzheimer's disease collaborative care model were published by our group at Indiana University and our friends at University of California at Los Angeles (UCLA). These crucial studies demonstrated the effectiveness of the collaborative care model in meeting the health needs of both the patients living with Alzheimer's disease and their unpaid caregivers.[8,9] Our model at IU was called PREVENT, which stood for Providing Resources Early to Vulnerable Elders Needing Treatment for Memory Loss. The model incorporated care by a multidisciplinary team led by a nurse practitioner who worked directly with the patients, the unpaid caregivers, and the primary care physicians. Furthermore, PREVENT utilized measurement-based and evidence-based care protocols to monitor and manage the cognitive, physical, and psychological disabilities of the patient as well as to support and coach their unpaid caregivers on problem solving strategies and effective coping skills.

PREVENT was tested over five years at the primary care practices within Eskenazi Health. UCLA's randomized controlled trial (conducted around the same time as the PREVENT trial) tested a very similar collaborative care model and produced similar results, confirming the effectiveness of the collaborative care model for Alzheimer's disease. Basically, these two studies demonstrated that if implemented properly, a collaborative care model could improve the behavioral and psychological disabilities of patients living with Alzheimer's disease while reducing the burden of the unpaid caregiver and thus improving the quality of care and quality of life for both the patient and the unpaid caregiver.[8,9] The studies' outcomes demonstrated that the collaborative care model results in:

- Improved quality of care for Alzheimer's disease
- Improved satisfaction with care
- Reduction in behavioral and psychological disabilities
- Reduction in unpaid caregiver distress and burden

It is hard to overstate how important these results were. Randomized controlled trials are the gold standard for demonstrating the efficacy of a clinical technique or treatment in order to receive approval by the federal government and subsequently have it covered by health insurance. The PREVENT study findings were published in one of the most prestigious peer-reviewed medical journals in the world, the *Journal of the American Medical Association.* As we will discuss in more detail later, when selecting effective solutions for healthcare delivery systems, one of the key components is to select evidence-based solutions. Each evidence-based solution is appropriately vetted, tested, and analyzed for consistency and viability within the healthcare environment. Eskenazi Health was fortunate enough to have two recently published studies to support the collaborative care model, establishing sufficient evidence to approve the program.

However, while we were confident that we had identified an effective and evidence-based model for Alzheimer's disease care, we also understood the challenges involved in implementing this model in the real world. Change is difficult, even when its intended benefits are clear. Each individual hospital and health system has its own culture and unique set of characteristics such as size, location, makeup, and patient population. In almost any setting, making a care delivery change is not simply a matter of rewriting policy or posting the steps of a new process. In addition to the variety of clinicians and staff (physicians, nurses, medical assistants, social workers, practice managers, lab techs, etc.), everyone has a unique set of skills, strengths, tendencies, and varying levels of experience. As unique individuals, we likely differ in our opinions, beliefs, outlooks, and attitudes. Despite these potential conflicts, all care providers and staff in a healthcare delivery organization must collaborate to provide the best possible care for patients. Changing a healthcare environment often means changing personal habits and the ways clinicians, administrators, and staff communicate with each other and their patients.

Too often, an organization can suffer from a culture that does not encourage the expression of new ideas and potential innovations from all levels of employees. Through all this adaptation, we must remember that we are asking for changes by individuals who are under tremendous levels of stress and have limited time to learn new processes or methods. People have a natural tendency to default to what is familiar and/or has worked for them previously, especially when under significant stress (as many healthcare environments seem to produce). When considering the complexity of the typical healthcare delivery system, it is easy to see why incorporating evidence-based solutions into real-world practice takes so long—or never occurs at all.

We needed to find a way to understand this complex system of individuals operating within a complex environment so that we could figure out how best to facilitate the change we knew was necessary and would ultimately improve patients' lives. Our team needed to understand this complex system of interconnected individuals if we were going to implement a culture conducive to the change we wanted to establish in our patients' lives. With that in mind, we set to work.

AGING BRAIN CARE MODEL

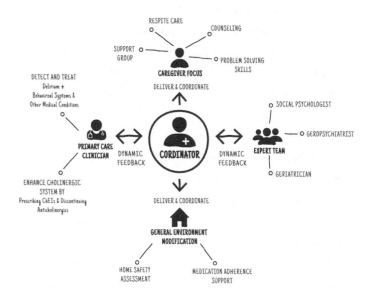

In September 2007, Lisa Harris, MD, the CEO of Eskenazi, a professor of medicine at Indiana University and a previous healthcare services researcher, confirmed the readiness of Eskenazi Health to address the gap in Alzheimer's care. In addition to the overwhelming evidence of the collaborative care model's ability to improve outcomes, a preliminary cost analysis provided early indications that the solution was both viable and sustainable at Eskenazi. Dr. Harris then challenged me, Dr. Callahan, and our colleagues at the Indiana University Center for Aging Research to convert the PREVENT model into a scalable and sustainable clinical program to be implemented within Eskenazi as soon as possible. The organization would provide full support of the design and implementation efforts, on one condition. The new clinic had to begin serving patients by January 2008. Converting the research model to an operating clinical program would require significant clinical practice redesign—and this work now had to be completed within four months!

What would ultimately become the Healthy Aging Brain Center (HABC) had its origins in that challenge, but the full manifestation of the HABC required significant effort. The first step was assembling a team of experts in Alzheimer's care including a primary care physician, three geriatricians, a nurse, a social worker, two neuropsychologists, a social psychologist, a clinic administrator, and a representative from the local Alzheimer's Association. The team was charged with identifying the minimum specifications necessary to deliver the care described in the PREVENT model. Despite their hectic schedules, the team committed to meeting biweekly. It would require diligent and consistent collaborative work to adapt the PREVENT model to the unique needs of patients while maintaining fidelity to the original intervention model. After 16 weeks, the team delivered seven minimum specifications of the new Alzheimer's care to Eskenazi leadership:

1. Patient and family caregiver education, coaching, and support
2. Periodic needs assessment and evaluation of an Alzheimer's care plan

3. Prevention and treatment of other brain conditions in the context of the presence of Alzheimer's disease such as delirium, depression, or anxiety

4. Medication management including describing effective medications, stopping (or de-prescribing) potentially harmful medications, and supporting patients' adherence to taking the right medications at the right time for the right dose

5. Management of vascular risk factors

6. Identification and management of excess disability due to other medical conditions that accompany Alzheimer's disease such as diabetes, heart failure, or infections

7. Coordination of care among diverse healthcare providers within the healthcare system and the entire community

The vision was to deliver the seven minimum specifications in two phases of care. The first phase would begin prior to the first appointment. To initiate the process, a care coordinator contacts the patient's unpaid caregiver by telephone to conduct a structured, comprehensive assessment of the patient's symptoms, functional status, medical history, and social situation as well as the unpaid caregiver's concerns and needs. During the first clinic visit, the physician would perform a complete diagnostic evaluation including a medical assessment, a structured physical and neurological examination, and both blood work and brain imaging as needed. In addition, the patients would be administered a battery of neuropsychological tests to measure their cognitive performance such as their short-term memory, language, and speed of processing information. After all test results were returned, the physician would make a diagnosis and the team would then develop an individualized brain care plan. At a later date, the patient would return, accompanied by family members, for a second appointment (family conference visit) where the physician and care coordinators would disclose the diagnosis, answer any questions, finalize the brain care plan with the patients, the unpaid caregiver, and the entire family, and initiate the execution of such a plan.

The second phase of care represents follow-up care. Follow-up care would be delivered both face-to-face in the clinic and by telephone. The frequency and type of follow-up would be dependent on the diagnosis, the brain care plan, the emergent needs of the patient and unpaid caregiver, and the preferences and goals of the patient and unpaid caregiver. Patients and unpaid caregivers would be encouraged to contact the care team in between visits whenever they had questions or needed assistance. During all follow-up contacts, the clinical team would assess both the patient and unpaid caregiver to identify cognitive, functional, behavioral, and psychological problems faced by the patient and the unpaid caregiver. In response to these assessments, the brain care plan would be modified to address changing needs and concerns.

The team felt these specifications addressed the needs of both the patients and their unpaid caregivers. They designed the phases to allow for iterative adjustment and to promote collaboration, coordination, and communication between patients, unpaid caregivers, and clinicians. Each patient received an individualized care plan, the details of which were carefully explained to the patient's unpaid caregivers. The team emphasized the need to discuss the scientific logic behind a plan's components to facilitate buy-in from the patient's caregivers.

Presenting the plan to patients and unpaid caregivers and allowing them to ask questions is more than just a transfer of information; it allows patients and their unpaid caregivers to be involved in the process, understand clinical decisions made, and provide input and feedback that may be unique to their loved one's situation. In a nutshell, the patient and the unpaid caregiver co-design the brain care plan with the clinical team. The ongoing review and revision of the care plan ensures that the individualized care continues to reflect not only what is best for that patient clinically, but also their desires and wishes and those of their unpaid caregivers. It is important to remember the family often faces difficult decisions regarding the type and intensity of the care provided to their loved one.

Once these seven minimum specifications were reviewed, discussed, and approved, Eskenazi leadership agreed on an evaluation plan to monitor outcomes during the first year. Performance metrics included a set of quality indicators as well as both ambulatory and acute care utilization. The plan also included a strategy to compare the performance of primary care centers delivering care for similar patients within the same time period.

Eskenazi announced the HABC via system-wide communications and several meetings with the primary care providers. On January 7, 2008 (within the deadline imposed by Dr. Harris), the clinic opened its doors with a ribbon-cutting ceremony attended by both hospital leadership and community stakeholders. A multidisciplinary team composed of a physician, two care coordinators (a registered nurse and a social worker), and a medical assistant began serving patients in three half-day clinics per week.

The team implementing the HABC understood that regular performance feedback loops are critical during implementation. They knew they needed to identify what was effective and what was not, while monitoring the program's impact on the system as a whole. In this case, the goal was to identify unintended consequences (or unintended benefits to leverage).

Throughout the various phases of the HABC implementation, a variety of performance feedback loops were utilized. During the design phase, the implementation team examined both clinical and cost data to understand:

1. the system's demand for Alzheimer's care services
2. potential revenue generated by the new program
3. potential cost savings associated with preventing inappropriate acute-care events

This data was used to garner additional support for the HABC from Eskenazi leadership. During the first year of the program, the implementation team monitored clinical outcomes and processes and adjusted care delivery along the way. The team collected assessment data from both patients and unpaid caregivers at every visit, tracked progress over time, and instituted needed modifications. Through process monitoring, several modifications became possible to the program, such as neuropsychological testing administration. Originally, a nurse and social worker shared responsibility for administering neuropsychological testing to new patients. Unfortunately, due to this responsibility, they were often unavailable to provide care coordination and counseling services in the clinic. When this conflict was identified, a new staff member was hired and trained to assume the testing role. Although this change increased the cost of the program, the team was able to see patients more efficiently and employee satisfaction improved.

ABC ANNUAL COST SAVINGS PER PATIENT

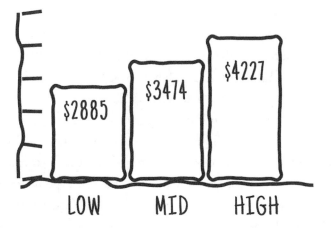

After one year, the implementation team reviewed clinical outcomes and performance metrics prescribed for the HABC by Eskenazi leadership. The clinical outcomes demonstrated effective disability management and a reduction in unpaid caregiver burden, both consistent with the results of the foundational PREVENT trial. Descriptive data revealed that depression was a comorbid condition for 55% of the patients seen in the HABC. In response, we provided additional staff training in the collaborative care model for depression. Other data from the first year of operations demonstrated cost savings achieved through reduced inpatient, emergency department, and related outpatient care expenditures.

The minimum specifications for the HABC were established during the design phase based on a comprehensive review of the PREVENT collaborative care model. After one year and several iterations, the day-to-day operations began to stabilize, were documented in a minimally standardized operating procedure, and were included in a manual designed to facilitate replication of the HABC.

In 2010, the HABC designed its own performance feedback loop with the development of the Enhanced Medical Record for Aging Brain Care (eMR-ABC), a web-based care coordination software. The eMR-ABC supports the user in the performance of both case management and population health management functions. The software calculates the measures and graphs trends over time. The user is thereby able to evaluate the performance of the entire population and quickly zoom in on the status of an individual patient and unpaid caregiver. Using this system, the clinical team can quickly identify all patients and unpaid caregivers with suboptimal outcomes and modify their plans of care to address areas of concern.

In the fall of 2015, Eskenazi announced plans to fund the new Sandra Eskenazi Center for Brain Care Innovation (CBCI), with the HABC as one of its flagship programs. CBCI has adopted the rather daunting vision of "Transforming brain health for all, now!" with an immediate goal of expanding high-quality Alzheimer's disease care services to meet the needs of more patients and unpaid caregivers. With that goal in mind, the HABC was asked to select a solution for scaling and spreading its services. After deliberation, once again the Agile Implementation model provided the blueprint to guide such an expansion.

A diverse team of providers, clinicians, and administrators in the HABC developed a plan that was subsequently approved by

STANDARDIZED MINIMUM AGING BRAIN CARE 2.0

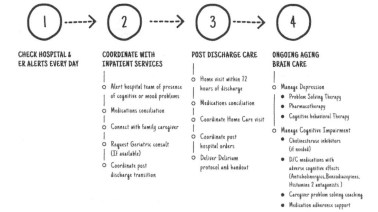

1	2	3	4
CHECK HOSPITAL & ER ALERTS EVERY DAY	COORDINATE WITH INPATIENT SERVICES	POST DISCHARGE CARE	ONGOING AGING BRAIN CARE

CHECK HOSPITAL & ER ALERTS EVERY DAY

COORDINATE WITH INPATIENT SERVICES
- Alert hospital team of presence of cognitive or mood problems
- Medications conciliation
- Connect with family caregiver
- Request Geriatric consult (IF available)
- Coordinate post discharge transition

POST DISCHARGE CARE
- Home visit within 72 hours of discharge
- Medications conciliation
- Coordinate Home Care visit
- Coordinate post hospital orders
- Deliver Delirium protocol and handout

ONGOING AGING BRAIN CARE
- Manage Depression
  - Problem Solving Therapy
  - Pharmacotherapy
  - Cognitive behavioral Therapy
- Manage Cognitive Impairment
  - Cholinesterase inhibitors (if needed)
  - D/C medications with adverse cognitive effects (Anticholinergics, Benzodiazepines, Histamine 2 antagonists)
  - Caregiver problem solving coaching
  - Medication adherence support

Eskenazi leadership. The plan (known as HABC 2.5) included several changes necessary to fully embrace the principles of population health management including:

1. Establishing panels of patients who will receive services from a collaborative care team, including a physician, social worker, and community health worker. Members of the team will serve the multidisciplinary needs of patients and unpaid caregivers across care settings (in the clinic as well as in the home);

2. Implementing new strategies for enrolling patients and unpaid caregivers and keeping them engaged;

3. Establishing a 24/7 Nurse HelpLine to assist patients and unpaid caregivers after hours with a goal of reducing unnecessary visits to the emergency room;

4. Partnering with scientists at Indiana University Center for Aging Research to develop and test new technologies that will allow care to be delivered in the space between the unpaid caregiver and a mobile device without the need for human intervention; and

5. Providing Alzheimer's care services pursuant to a contract with a managed care insurer or accountable care organization.

Lessons Learned

Looking back, I can see that the crucial challenge of the HABC was not finding an effective and evidence-based care model; both studies used to support the initiative were readily available. Instead, the challenge was in operationalizing and implementing the model into an existing practice where the team faced most of its obstacles. We were able to triumph over that challenge because we utilized a process of implementation that acknowledged both the complexity of the health system and the uniqueness of the individuals within. We know now that this difficulty in implementation is a common theme across the healthcare landscape, and this challenge became a driving force behind what ultimately became the Agile Implementation model.

Chapter 2

Caring for the Survivors
of Critical Illness:
The ICU Survivorship Clinic

very year in the US more than five million patients
are admitted to intensive care units (ICU) around
the country.[10] The number is staggering and will only
grow as our population ages and life expectancies improve.
Typically, when a patient visits the ICU, they are facing a life-
threatening illness and often endure complicated and invasive
treatments to keep them alive. The good news is that due to
advances in this area of medical care, patients are more likely
to survive their ICU visit than ever before.[11] The bad news,
however, is that for those who survive, the stress of their
illness and the invasive treatments they endured often leave

them suffering from cognitive, physical, and/or psychological disabilities. These might include depression, anxiety, and even post-traumatic stress disorder, as well as cognitive impairment and physical weakness.

These conditions can have a profound effect on patients' health and quality of life going forward. Fatigue and weakness stemming from neuropathy can make it difficult to participate in activities or social situations that previously felt effortless. Patients may find it difficult to return to work (or may require a significant delay before they are able to), complete household tasks, or manage their medications and their own finances. Studies have found that in some cases, the detriment to quality of life can persist for up to five years after they are discharged from the ICU.[12]

To better understand what was happening within our own facility, we conducted a natural history study. It was late 2010, and we studied a population of 1,149 patients who were admitted to Eskenazi Health's medical-surgical ICU between May 2009 and May 2010. The only other criterion we used for this patient population was to focus on those who had survived their critical illness and their stay at the ICU for at least 30 days. When we looked at the results, we saw that 37% of the ICU survivors suffered from acute lung injury or delirium (acute brain failure) during their ICU stay, both serious and dangerous conditions. When we followed those patients forward, 36% of those with acute lung injury and 48% of those with delirium were hospitalized again in the subsequent 11 months. Additionally, about one out of every 20 of those with acute lung injury and

37%

OF ICU SURVIVORS
SUFFER FROM
ACUTE LUNG INJURY
OR DELIRIUM

ICU Survivors
Over 11 months
-------->

OF THOSE WITH
ACUTE LUNG-INJURY

4% **36%**
DIED HOSPITALIZED

OF THOSE
WITH DELIRIUM

13% **48%**
DIED HOSPITALIZED

Source: Khan BA1, Lasiter S, Boustani MA. CE: critical care recovery center: an innovative collaborative care model for ICU survivors. Am J Nurs. 2015 Mar;115(3):24-31; quiz 34, 46. doi: 10.1097/01.NAJ.0000461807.42226.3e.

about one out of every 8 with delirium died during that same period.

It was clear to us and to the hospital's leadership that improving care and outcomes for this population was a priority. Additionally, key stakeholders of Eskenazi noted trends within the larger healthcare environment highlighting the need for improved care of these patients. Specifically, it was becoming more common for hospitals to care for critically ill patients, as opposed to those with lesser conditions or simply chronic diseases like hypertension or diabetes. Several administrators took notice of this trend and saw high-quality post-ICU care as a marketable attribute of the facility. This was also a time when federal reimbursement systems (Medicare and Medicaid) began to hold hospitals accountable for the care of patients for a period of time after their initial hospital discharge. In the years to come, multiple federal quality reporting programs would begin to measure the rates of hospital readmission within 30 days. Those hospitals that fared worse relative to their peers would face potential financial penalties in the form of lower reimbursement. So, in addition to improving care for patients surviving the ICU, there was a significant business case to be made that confirmed demand within the institution for a solution to the issue of designing care for the ICU survivors.

To address this need, we created the Critical Care Recovery Center (CCRC) with a goal of providing collaborative care to ICU survivors.[13] The first step in the CCRC's creation was to gather an interdisciplinary team from the critical care and geriatrics divisions at the Indiana University School of Medicine who had used collaborative care models for patients with dementia, depression, and other geriatric syndromes. Many on this team had previously developed research protocols and research tools to meet the complex recovery needs of ICU survivors and found themselves tasked with how to transfer their research discoveries into a clinical delivery process within the CCRC.

Initially, we used the HABC as a model for the CCRC. The HABC had demonstrated a positive impact on the care of patients and unpaid caregivers living with Alzheimer's disease within its first years of existence, and we felt it provided an efficient model for how to structure the CCRC. Brainstorming sessions and deliberations regarding the CCRC's structure and functioning started well in advance of its opening. We held quarterly meetings in 2010 and 2011 to discuss strategy, using the same Agile Implementation process. The meetings involved all stakeholders: leadership from Indiana University School of Medicine's critical care and geriatrics divisions; the Indiana University Center for Aging Research; and critical care nursing, physical rehabilitation, and neuropsychology departments. Through these meetings the stakeholders recognized and codified the vision for improving the cognitive, physical, and psychological outcomes of ICU survivors. The meetings also provided the time and space for the stakeholders to develop relationships, reflect on the challenges, and identify the minimum specifications for the CCRC. Potential members were identified for the smaller operational teams that would meet weekly to solve problems, monitor progress, and—once the program launched in July 2011—make timely modifications based on incoming data.

The delivery team identified four minimum specifications for the CCRC regarding patient care:

1. Maximize full cognitive, physical, and psychological recovery following hospitalization for a critical illness
2. Enhance patient and family caregiver satisfaction
3. Improve the quality of transitional and rehabilitation care
4. Reduce unnecessary hospitalizations and ED visits

To identify the minimum specifications for the CCRC, we leveraged guidelines and evidence-based protocols already in existence to identify crucial aspects such as: performing an early assessment of functionality, providing patient and unpaid caregiver education and coaching, and monitoring health outcomes longitudinally. However, we had to adapt these concepts to the local environment to be used by the CCRC.

To translate components of the evidence-based protocol locally and to meet the cognitive, functional, and psychological needs of ICU survivors and their family caregivers, we employed multiple "sprints." Sprints are short, intense cycles of implementation where components are put into practice to see how they perform and function at the local level. After a sprint, staff provide feedback regarding their experience and discuss potential adjustments they feel would make the process more effective and sustainable. Appropriate modifications are made before the next sprint, and this iterative process continues until all are satisfied that the component is at its most effective for the local environment and intended use. As an example, during one of the first sprints we observed high rates of no-shows to the first CCRC visit. This reflected the lack of an adequate link between ICU discharge and subsequent care through the CCRC. To address this, we added a direct referral from the ICU for 90 days after discharge and set up a pre-clinic phone call with patients and their unpaid caregivers. The purpose was to make sure they understood the benefits the CCRC could provide them. We immediately saw a drop in the rate of no-shows.

In addition to performing sprints to localize the critical components, the team also needed to measure and track the CCRC performance and its impact on the system as a whole. Just as with the HABC, the team understood that changes implemented through the CCRC could influence care and outcomes across the health system, and this impact needed monitoring. To do this, the team distributed quarterly dashboards with data on several measures, including the percent receiving antidepressants and the number of primary care or specialty visits patients had. The dashboards also allowed the team to evaluate changes in cognitive, functional, behavioral, and psychological disabilities at multiple time points. To assess system impact, the team tracked overall readmissions, ED use, and a variety of costs related to care utilization.

Now finalized, the collaborative care team of the CCRC consists of a nurse, a critical care physician, a social worker, a medical assistant, and a technician, with support services from physical therapy, neuropsychology, and psychiatry. Currently, both the nurse and social worker function as care coordinators. Clinic nurses manage the flow of the clinic, lead family conferences, oversee medication reconciliation, conduct scheduling and follow-up phone calls, and partner with the designated unpaid caregivers to coach them on stress reduction techniques and coping skills. A pharmacist is available for consultation about drug management, as needed.

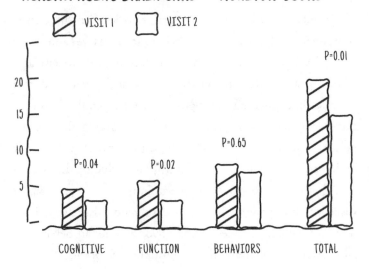

HEALTHY AGING BRAIN CARE — MONITOR SCORE

MINIMALLY STANDARD CARE

 Support for **early and accurate** rehabilitation of patients' cognitive, physical and psychological functions

 Support for patient and family **education** and counseling to activate self-rehabilitation

 Support for clinical decision-making to accomplish targeted rehabilitation goals including steps to consider with initial treatment failure

 Support for longitudinal **monitoring** of patient outcomes and coordinate care

 Support for an effective **medication prescribing** process including discontinuing inappropriate medications, reconcile medication regimens and enhancing medication adherence

 Timely access to specialty **consultation,** co-management or specialty care

Early results of the CCRC demonstrated improvements in cognitive, functional, and behavioral measures and a reduction in acute healthcare utilization.[13]

The program is currently in its eighth year of operation. The development of a minimally standardized operating procedure allowed the service to be adapted for home-based ICU survivors and trauma survivors. With support from the National Institute on Aging, our scientific team is currently evaluating the impact of using a home-based and scalable version of the CCRC program model in meeting the needs of patients who are unable to attend the clinics and those who have survived surgical trauma.

Lesson Learned

Just as with the HABC, the development of the CCRC was born from a need to improve care for a select group of patients in a setting where there was already evidence-based guidance on what that care should look like. While the physicians recognized a need for improvement in care, administrators confirmed demand for change by recognizing the opportunity to improve the entire organization. Along with our experiences developing the HABC, the process of creating the CCRC allowed us to identify the key aspects of successful and sustainable implementations. More importantly, we were beginning to understand *why* these aspects were so instrumental in the success and sustainability of solutions. The observations we made during the HABC would ultimately allow us to develop a model applicable to any type of care in any setting. It was an exciting time, and while we were close to developing the model that would become the Agile Implementation model, we still had some things to learn.

Chapter 3

Reducing Central Line-Associated Bloodstream Infections

The sun was shining through the hospital room window on what promised to be an exciting day. After five months of fighting cancer, Mr. Smith was getting ready to receive his sixth and final round of chemotherapy through a Central Line. Mr. Smith had grown fond of these Central Lines, the plastic tubes placed in his arm that traveled his veins all the way to his heart. He had learned how to take care of them, ensuring they were clean and dry. In return, these Central Lines were taking care of him. They delivered the chemotherapy to his blood, allowed the nurses to draw blood without having to stick him with a needle, and delivered any medicines or blood products to make him feel better. Mr. Smith and the Central

Lines enjoyed a close and vital relationship. Meticulously changed, maintained, and replaced every month, they might even have been considered close friends.

When his doctor came into the room, Mr. Smith could not hold back his excitement. This was his last chemotherapy before returning to his normal life. He had a good chance to survive his cancer, and his doctor quoted him a 75% chance that the cancer would never return. Mr. Smith was optimistic, sharing his post-recovery plans with his physician. Mr. Smith had worked hard all his life, and now, at the age of 66, he had retired to spend time traveling with his wife to all the destinations they had dreamed of visiting. He also was looking forward to having time to make memories with his grandchildren and being a greater presence in their lives. His doctor was happy for him, thinking to himself, *My life is so meaningful. I am so fortunate to help people who are suffering overcome their cancer and go back to making their dreams come true!*

Four days later, Mr. Smith started feeling weak and had chills. Although he was due to leave the hospital after the last chemotherapy infusion through his Central Line the next day, he didn't have the energy to celebrate. All he wanted to do was lie in bed. Then he developed a fever. The chills became more intense. He was exhausted. His wife was getting concerned; he was paler than usual. The nurses came into his room telling him they had to get "blood cultures" to diagnose the fever; he might have an infection. Later the doctors came in and told him that his blood pressure was getting low and they needed to take him to the intensive care unit. Mr. Smith was feeling so weak he could not stay awake. By the next morning he was unconscious and the doctors had to place him on artificial life support because his organs were failing. His wife was terrified, asking herself, "Is he going to die?"

A few days later, the doctors asked to meet with the family. Sadness and fear weighed heavy in the room. The doctors somberly shared that Mr. Smith's Central Line had become infected and spread that infection to his blood. In turn, his body was at its most vulnerable against the malady and his organs had failed. "He is not going to make it," they said. "We should not prolong his suffering." Everyone was crying and wondering, *How could this happen?! The Central Line that was helping him receive his lifesaving treatment is now taking his life. Is this real?*

Hospital-acquired infections, or HAIs, have garnered a tremendous amount of attention over the last several years— as well they should, because these are infections that patients obtained *after* they were admitted to the hospital. Perhaps most importantly, these infections are sometimes preventable. Among the most common types of HAIs are those due to the presence of Central Lines. These Central Line-associated bloodstream infections, or CLABSIs, occur in an estimated 80,000 patients a year,[14,15] cost hundreds of millions of dollars a year to treat,[14] and are potentially life-threatening. Additionally, they are often included in quality monitoring programs where facilities can face financial penalties if their CLABSI rates are too high.

As with other conditions, evidence-based guidelines have been published and "prevention bundles" (groups of procedures and policies intended to reduce the risk of infection) have been developed but have not been fully implemented in facilities around the country.[16] Similar to the circumstances around the care for patients living with Alzheimer's disease and those who survived critical illness, evidence-based guidelines and solutions are readily available. As we have learned through the previous studies, the challenge is not in identifying the effective treatment; the challenge is figuring out how to take the evidence-based solutions and apply them to the complex and unique environment within an individual facility.

In 2015, facing many of the same pressures regarding HAIs as other facilities nationwide, the leadership at the Indiana University Health Adult Academic Health Centers identified CLABSI reduction as the highest safety priority for their facility in 2016. The Health Centers consist of two adult tertiary care hospitals in Indianapolis with approximately 1,100 licensed beds and 36,000 annual admissions. As with many urban health centers, the patient population is diverse in background, ethnicity, and socio-economic status. Key stakeholders understood the implications for CLABSI reduction and knew that improvement in this area meant patients like Mr. Smith could return to their normal lives without the fear of an infection from their Central Line.

Those within the Academic Health Centers charged with developing, implementing, and sustaining this change knew that it would require multiple steps and rely heavily on staff from several departments to cooperate and function in concert. In response, an interdisciplinary team of providers met several times in early 2016 to try to adapt existing practice guidelines for preventing catheter-related infections and evidence-based recommendations for reducing CLABSI to the local environment.

PROCESS TO REDUCE CLABSIS

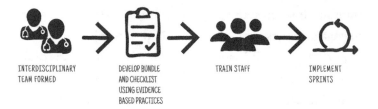

INTERDISCIPLINARY
TEAM FORMED

DEVELOP BUNDLE
AND CHECKLIST
USING EVIDENCE
BASED PRACTICES

TRAIN STAFF

IMPLEMENT
SPRINTS

During these sessions, this diverse team of physicians, nurses, pharmacists, and infection preventionists established a set of localized practice guidelines, created a maintenance bundle checklist, and developed training curriculum for the providers and staff. The guidelines specified the indications for Central Line placement, removal, duration, and the type of line to be used. The bundle included daily chlorhexidine gluconate bathing, appropriate dressing, tubing changes, skin care, and hub disinfection. A checklist served as a reminder for ensuring that the dressing was clean, dry, and occlusive, as well as for encouraging the use of appropriate steps when it became necessary to change dressing and tubing. In congruence with the bundle, the team developed a training curriculum aimed at improving multiple aspects of care, including bundle adherence as stipulated by the guidelines, sterile technique with line placement, hand hygiene, and central line maintenance. The team designed the training as an interprofessional collaborative effort, incorporating input from providers with expertise in line insertion and care, and focused on improving interactions among semiautonomous agents from different professions and disciplines.

The interdisciplinary team knew as well as anyone that simply having the information would not be enough to ensure that staff followed the checklist or even attended the training. To address this, significant time and effort was spent to engage leaders at multiple levels in the organization, as well as key staff and clinicians. With their attention, it was easier to raise awareness about the problem and motivate buy-in at multiple levels of hierarchy. The team used storytelling and other methods to appeal to the hearts and minds of those they needed to engage. Resulting from their efforts, demand for the training was established and likelihood was increased that staff would attend and advocate for others to join as well. These efforts paid dividends. Between February and September 2016 this curriculum was presented to more than 300 physicians and 1,000 nurses. New staff also received this training, including first-year residents and fellows who were expected to insert central lines. This training is still ongoing (2019) and has since enrolled more than 1,000 new physicians and interns. The training was never mandatory, even though other leaders thought it should be. But the Safety and Infection Prevention leadership knew that internally motivated clinicians are much more passionate and willing than those whose attendance is forced.

In June 2016, the medical directors and nursing managers of all units with high rates of CLABSI convened to begin implementation sprints of the localized solution. Along with the Quality/Safety and Infection Prevention teams, these parties met every two weeks to review CLABSI events in their units and discuss the top three implementation challenges they faced (to provide learnings for subsequent sprints). At each meeting, representatives from each unit addressed the following:

1. What did you do that worked well?
2. What did not work well?
3. What do you plan to do differently based on what you learned?

This process facilitated communication between units and fostered a sense of shared accountability across the Academic Health Centers. Between meetings to monitor the success of implementation, units employed visual tools such as scoreboards and charts to engage frontline staff and track their progress. When a unit struggled with performance, staff leveraged quality resources to observe the environment and understand factors influencing performance. Among the factors noted, the most common were behavioral triggers, attitudes and beliefs, habits, processes, networks, and interpersonal relationships, as well as organizational facilitators and barriers.

Specifically, staff used the skills of the Infection Prevention specialists and clinical nurse specialists assigned to each unit and reviewed data from clinical dashboards to identify areas for improvement. These findings were discussed at the meetings, and the best practice units supported plans for improvement.

The team understood from the evidence-based guidelines and recommendations that there were clear metrics that could be used to evaluate success and sustainability of the employed solution and monitor the impact on the system as a whole. These included the incidence rate per days at risk, Central

CLABSI INCIDENCE RATE

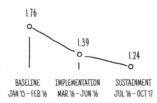

CAUTI INCIDENCE RATE

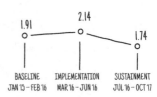

C-DIFF INCIDENCE RATE

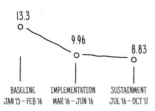

TOTAL HARMS PER MONTH

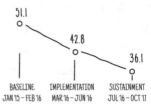

	BASELINE JAN '15 – FEB '16	IMPLEMENTATION MAR '16 – JUN '16	SUSTAINMENT JUL '16 – OCT '17
CLABSI INCIDENCE RATE	1.76	1.39	1.24
CAUTI INCIDENCE RATE	1.91	2.14	1.74
C-DIFF INCIDENCE RATE	13.3	9.96	8.83
TOTAL HARMS PER MONTH	51.1	42.8	36.1

Abbreviations: CLABSI, Central-Line Associated Blood Stream Infection; CAUTI, Catheter-Associated Urinary Tract Infection; C-Diff, Clostridium Difficile

Line utilization, and the rate of compliance with the Central Line bundle. The team also understood that CLABSIs are just one type of infection, and infections are just one type of patient harm. It was reasonable to assume that efforts to reduce CLABSIs could potentially spill over into other areas and produce unforeseen improvements. It was also possible, however, that intense focus on CLABSIs could lead to other infections and patient harms receiving less attention, potentially resulting in increased rates of these other events. In short, the team knew that implementation to improve Central Line care would likely have an impact in other aspects of the health system, and it was crucial that they track measures that would allow them to evaluate and monitor that impact. Therefore, in addition to tracking the rate of CLABSI, the team also tracked rates of other HAIs, including catheter-associated urinary tract infections (CAUTIs), surgical site infections (SSIs) after abdominal hysterectomy and colon surgery, and Clostridium difficile (c-diff) infections. Additionally, overall harm events—comprised of the previously listed events along with falls resulting in injury, hospital acquired pressure ulcers, medication errors, serious medical errors, and mortality—were also measured.

Implementation occurred during a four-month period in 2016, from March through June. In addition to data from prior to the implementation period, the team tracked data for 14 months after the implementation period, from July 2016 through October 2017, which provided the opportunity to establish the sustainability of the implementation over the course of the intervention.

Ultimately, the intervention was successful at reducing CLABSIs. The incidence rate dropped by more than 50% from 1.76 infections per 1,000 central line days prior to the implementation to 0.78/1,000 days over the sustainment period, with the average number of CLABSIs per month being cut in half: from 12 per month to only six per month. Additionally, the team observed reductions in the rates of other infections, such as SSIs, over the same time period, while CAUTIs remained stable.[17]

The team and hospital administrators were thrilled with these results. It is important to remember that using the evidence-based solutions that were already available created these measures. That is, the success realized at the Academic Health Centers was not because of a new solution for Central Line maintenance and care, but because of how previously established guidelines and recommendations were implemented using adjustments for an environment with its own unique characteristics. There were clear reasons why *this* implementation was successful while countless previous attempts struggled to accomplish the same (or at least very similar) processes for reducing CLABSIs.

Wisely, those involved in this implementation sought feedback from the physicians and nurses to understand why this intervention found such sustainable success. Near the end of this project, staff were given an opportunity to offer their insight into the main drivers of success at a debriefing session. From this session and other feedback received, it became clear that a key driver of the success and sustainability of the solution was the increase in the engagement of physicians, nurses, and other clinical staff in the process of safety improvement and infection prevention. Additionally, staff talked about the favorable shift in the culture regarding patient-safety events. The punitive attitude toward these types of events that existed before the implementation had evolved into a more team-focused environment bent on shared learning and collaboratively improving care quality.

These changes in the interpersonal interactions within the healthcare system allowed and encouraged the improvement in care and confirmed what we had seen in our other activities: healthcare systems are complex in their composition and in the interactions of their members. Understanding these sources of variation and leveraging them for positive change was a powerful force. This complexity, in our opinion, also helps to explain the improvements in the rate of the other types of patient harms. We know that staff interact with providers from all parts of the facility, not just those within their department or center. It is reasonable to speculate that as a spillover effect of the intervention, the increase in communication and change in the overall safety culture regarding CLABSIs influenced the care and culture surrounding other areas of patient care.

Lessons Learned

One of the main takeaways from the CLABSI-reduction project was the notion that the intervention potentially had an impact on behavior and care delivery across the system and for a variety of patient harms. Again, it's impossible to know from our data how much of the change in other areas was due to the CLABSI reduction effort. It is true that certain rates of infections fell during the same period as implementation of the CLABSI standards; we were not able to prove relation in the events. However, if they were linked, it provides stunning insight. We observed how healthcare system members are unique individuals who use personal experiences and beliefs to respond in a situation, and when interacting with each other, that unique perspective compounds with each consulted staff in varying levels of complex interactions.

Any successful intervention will be one that not only allows for that complexity, but also embraces and leverages it to achieve the largest possible positive impact. Interventions that consider individual facility departments or divisions as independent silos of activity and personnel are less likely to be effective or sustainable. Because of the nature of healthcare systems, changes in procedure or processes will reverberate throughout the system, and in turn, the system as a whole will shape and influence the intervention and both its sustainability and success.

Part II
THEORIES AND FRAMEWORKS

The experiences described in the previous chapters represent thousands of hours of work and collaboration between dozens of dedicated professionals. The challenge of implementing beneficial and evidence-based innovations is not due to the lack of commitment or dedication of the amazing workforce of our healthcare delivery system, but rather to the complexity of the systems in which they interact. The delivery of high-quality patient care—effective and efficient assessments, accurate and appropriate treatment, thorough and compassionate communication—requires the seamless integration of complex systems and semiautonomous but interconnected individuals. Predicting or influencing decisions is difficult because individuals are remarkably unique and continuously develop their opinions and skillsets throughout their careers.

Additionally, internal and external pressures on time, money, and resources often influence the type of interactions clinical providers have with each other and their patients. When we consider the challenge of enabling change, we must remember that evidence-based solutions are often created and tested in controlled settings or within specific patient populations. Implementers can sometimes find it difficult to adapt these tailored approaches to meet the needs of a specific facility or system, especially if variables differ between the populations or circumstances the original solution applied to.

Over the course of several years and a myriad of interventions, we came to understand the need for a model of implementation that: (1) allowed for the complex nature of the healthcare delivery system; (2) acknowledged the uniqueness of the setting and individuals who worked there; and (3) leveraged an assortment of interactions of those individuals. To accomplish this, we examined previously established theories and frameworks of human behavior and system dynamics. The concepts we uncovered and distilled represent the building blocks of the Agile Implementation model and contains the theoretic explanation for why the model is successful in creating rapid, scalable, and sustainable change.

Chapter 4

Behavioral Economics

T he care received in a hospital or healthcare setting is largely (if not wholly in some cases) dependent on the decisions of individual healthcare providers. This suggests that our ability to improve the quality of care becomes a function of our ability to influence decisions and actions within the unique circumstances of a healthcare encounter. However, we also know that the individuals providing care are operating within a larger organization and in a specific care environment. As such, the process of care delivery is also a function of providers' interactions with other individuals and the physical infrastructure around them. Seen as a whole, each healthcare delivery system mixes cultural, social, and physical dynamics that a provider must consider when deliberating a decision. These systems exist as collaboration between multiple individuals pursuing a mission of patient care exceeding what they might accomplish individually.

These days, we have options for collaboration that did not exist for our ancestors. The establishment of the internet and advances in global travel have allowed for experts around the world to share information and results with remarkable speed. Individuals have greater agility in their ability to join in complex systems and organizations, even across international lines. However, the information of these multifaceted social groups did not begin with the internet. Humankind has sought and built these complex systems throughout our history. The statement "The whole is greater than the sum of its parts" reflects an important philosophy among the coalitions, centers, and other social systems on the cumulative effects of contribution. We recognize the power in cooperation, we can measure its efficacy in accomplishing goals, and we can note the ways these associations develop as entities.

As a complex social organization grows, it loses resemblance to the characteristics of individuals within and begins to take on its own unique identity. In his book *Scale: The Universal Laws of Life, Growth, and Death in Organisms, Cities, and Companies*, Geoffrey West observes that the "...dynamics, growth, and organization of animals, plants, human social behavior, cities, and companies are, in fact, subject to similar generic laws." Regardless of the scale between individual and organization, both can be observed, their development predicted, and their behavior influenced by comparable methods. As we will explore, an understanding of these complex systems and their dynamics will provide specific strategies for how to influence human behavior to achieve a desired change. Within the constructs of such a system, outcomes are dictated not only by complex dynamics, but also by choices and actions of individual members. Interactions with other members and the physical environment, in turn, influence these choices and actions. We must also remember that at the core of these elements is an ever-changing individual who subjects each solution to his or her unique characteristics. Therefore, understanding how complex systems function requires an examination of individual behaviors and the forces that can influence personal decisions to become actions.

When it comes to examining, explaining, and even predicting individual behavior, the field of behavioral economics has made substantial discoveries over the last several decades. As its name implies, behavioral economics was originally pursued to explain why consumers make certain decisions related to economic activities such as purchasing, saving, and investing. Some decisions you may be familiar with include why does offering a "free trial" or "money-back guarantee" increase the likelihood of purchase? Or why do sales of a product go up after a more expensive version of the same product is released into the market?

Eventually, social scientists began to apply the concepts of behavioral economics to situations outside of economic markets or consumerism in an attempt to refine the logic of human behavior. Questions such as why the location of foods in the school lunch line influence the likelihood of their selection, or why the offer of a financial incentive increases smoking cessation rates are just two of the behaviors scientists hoped to explain. These examples are natural extensions of the original concepts because, at their heart, is a desire to uncover a deeper insight. Namely, *how do people evaluate options and decide which one to pursue?* We all encounter daily circumstances where our evaluation is tested, and we must quickly come to a decision. Often, the subsequent decisions and actions can influence social interactions, monetary gains or losses, and even our health. Understanding these basic mental processes provides a glimpse into a more fundamental understanding of what it means to be human and to live and react in a social and interconnected environment.

Behavioral economics can be considered an integration of economics and social science principles stemming from sociology, psychology, and neuroscience. In contrast to traditional economics, which is based on the assumptions that people will wisely choose between alternatives, behavioral economics recognizes the concept of 'bounded rationality'.[18] The idea states that humans' ability to make rational decisions is limited by a multitude of factors; the type and amount of information available at the time of decision and the amount of time available are examples of facets that limit one's understanding of a situation and its potential implications. This concept advocates that behavioral decisions are not consistently rational but rather strongly influenced by an interplay of cognitive, emotional, and social forces.[19] Stated differently, the individuals who make decisions are shaped by and embedded within social environments. Interactions with the external and internal stressors of a situation along with personal attributes often inform the behavior of individuals and subsequently the networks they inhabit. Relational attributes between people such as empathy, trust, and shared experiences are as effective at influencing decisions and behavior as personal attributes like emotion, attention, and skills.

As they apply to the delivery of healthcare, these concepts explain the forces at work during a typical healthcare encounter. During an initial patient encounter, the provider must make a decision about appropriate care under the auspices of bounded rationality. Limitations in available time, information, and understanding can often impede any decision regarding both the patient and their condition. The provider may be impacted by personal attributes such as their current level of stress or workload, their capacity to empathize, and their ability to unearth the true nature of the patient's illness or discomfort. Clearly, the provider's decisions and actions (as well as those of his or her colleagues) are also a function of the social and cultural environment in which he or she works every day. The current interaction exhibits no independence from the other interactions that have occurred leading up to that point. For example, if a provider has recently learned of an increase in measles in the surrounding community, it may be at the forefront of their mind when they encounter a patient who presents with a fever, sore throat, and eye irritation. Although these symptoms are common to measles, they could also easily be attributed to other maladies and perhaps lead to a hasty and erroneous diagnosis.

At first blush, you might say that all this variability stemming from social dynamics and individual uniqueness poses a problem in establishing a consistent system for the delivery of high-quality and high-value care. While true in one sense, the implication of these discoveries is actually quite positive. The revelation emerging from this understanding of human behavior is that *there exist opportunities to leverage information processing and decision making to encourage the desired outcome.* Specifically, it is possible to modify the social and physical environment to directly influence behavior. This is key. We posited previously that our ability to evoke change and improvement in healthcare delivery is a function of our ability to affect individuals' decisions and actions. The concepts gleaned from the work of behavioral economists, then, offer results for this endeavor, as long as we can figure out *how* to modify the social and physical environment to foster the desired change in behavior.

To achieve these results, we need to understand how individuals process and react to change. That is, we have established that individual attributes, personal interactions, and the physical environment can influence behavior, but we have not yet examined how that happens.

Certain theories[20,21] suggest that two types of cognitive processes govern individuals' behavior in response to environmental stimuli: one that is automatic and intuitive and another that is reflective and rational. The automatic system (sometimes referred to as System 1) is typically fast, requiring little effort or "thinking," while the reflective system (System 2) can be thought of as deliberate, slow, and requiring some

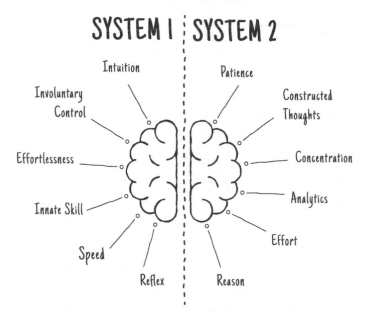

SYSTEM 1 : SYSTEM 2

Intuition

Patience

Involuntary Control

Constructed Thoughts

Effortlessness

Concentration

Innate Skill

Analytics

Speed

Effort

Reflex : Reason

level of mental effort.[19] As an example, while driving you likely utilize the reflective system to think about how you're going to get to your destination, but if another car unexpectedly swerved out in front of your car you would use your automatic system to quickly determine what immediate actions were necessary to avoid a collision.

The automatic system is not only used in the case of emergencies but as an initial reaction to almost any situation or stimulus. In most situations, you will have an initial reaction to information that is presented—the automatic system is quick and requires little mental effort. When told the cost to fix your furnace you are likely to have an immediate reaction as to whether the cost is reasonable. You are also likely to make an immediate judgment when asked to attend a movie based on whether you have any preexisting opinions about the particular film or genre. Keep in mind that your automatic system will make an evaluation regardless of how much (or how little) information it has.

In contrast, applying your reflective system requires you to expend the mental effort considering the details of the situation to arrive at a solution. A reflective choice is a *deliberation* taken to arrive at a conclusion while an automatic choice is a *reaction* based on the relevant information you have in that instant. Considering how differently these two cognitive processes function, it is not surprising that they frequently result in very different evaluations and interpretations. Although contrary to what you might think, neither system is completely problematic. Our life creates many situations in which instant reactions can be just as valuable as thoughtful deliberations. Problems tend to arise when one system is favored over another, or the *reaction* of an automatic system is not crosschecked by the *deliberation* of the reflective system. The automatic system arrives at an evaluation so quickly by reducing (i.e., filtering and discarding much of) the information it considers. Therefore, when making decisions based on this reduced information, the automatic process often relies on generalizations or rules of thumb that may or may not be accurate.

The pivotal breakthrough in this theory was explored in a series of works by Amos Tversky and Daniel Kahneman from the 1970s and beyond. Both carried out a series of experiments intended to reveal how people make decisions when presented with different scenarios or choices. In each test, subjects did not have complete information on which to base their evaluations, allowing observation of their reflective system decisions. The researchers identified several cognitive biases or "heuristics" inherent in the automatic process developed to filter excessive amounts of information. For example, in a "representativeness" bias, individuals compare whatever they are evaluating to a preconceived impression or mental picture (e.g., does the combination of symptoms this patient displays match my mental model of those with disease X?). Another heuristic identified was the "availability" bias suggesting that situations or outcomes more easily remembered by an individual are more likely to be believed (e.g., we just had someone in our waiting room with this disease; perhaps this is another case). Our human nature is embedded with biases, and several examples are included in the table below.

The concepts examined by Tversky and Kahneman (as well as others) not only identify and explain these biases but also provide a template for creating choice architectures, or

EXAMPLES OF EMBEDDED BIASES

MESSENGER
WE ARE HEAVILY INFLUENCED BY WHO DELIVERS INFORMATION

INCENTIVES
OUR RESPONSES TO INCENTIVES ARE SHAPED BY PREDICTABLE MENTAL SHORTCUTS SUCH AS STRONGLY AVOIDING LOSS

NORMS
WE ARE STRONGLY IMPACTED BY OUR PERCEPTION OF WHAT OTHERS ARE DOING

DEFAULTS
WE GO WITH THE FLOW AND TEND NOT TO CHANGE PRESET OPTIONS

SALIENCE
WE ARE DRAWN TO INFORMATION PERCEIVED TO BE NOVEL AND RELEVANT

PRIMING
WE ARE IMPACTED SUBCONSCIOUSLY BY ENVIRONMENTAL CUES

AFFECT
WE GO WITH OUR GUT FEELINGS; OUR FIRST, EMOTIONAL REACTION

COMMITMENTS
WE SEEK TO BE CONSISTENT WITH OUR PUBLIC PROMISES

EGO
WE WANT TO FEEL GOOD ABOUT OURSELVES

"nudges," that leverage human tendencies in information processing and behavior. Revisiting our previous examples, we know that providing a "free trial" induces people to try (and often keep) a product or service. They define the phenomenon as loss aversion: the tendency of consumers to value something more if they already possess it. We also know that placing fruits and vegetables at certain positions in the lunch line can influence schoolchildren to select those more often (and fewer sweets or desserts) because of heuristics related to availability and framing.

Not only is there information on how and why these nudges are effective, but it is also possible to determine when they might be most impactful to use. Nudges are most successful in situations where feedback on implicated results is not immediate or when we cannot draw upon sufficient knowledge or experience. The schoolchildren could benefit from a nudge to help make healthy eating choices. Many of us could use a nudge reminding us to contribute to our retirement savings as we tend to go without feedback on our account's adequacy until we need it.

Within a healthcare delivery setting, these concepts apply to numerous circumstances. We can infer how a choice architecture could *nudge* providers toward certain behaviors by leveraging their inherent bias. Some observable examples may include the following:

1. Altering the physical environment can change behavior; such adjustments can encourage certain interactions and the likelihood that certain actions will occur.

2. Who delivers information influences its impact; select a credible source or thought leader when communicating a change to peers.

3. Loss aversion is stronger than gain seeking; when considering incentives, a reward system is less effective than a loss avoidance system.

4. Availability of personal experiences can influence the perceived likelihood of events; if trying to avoid certain adverse events, remind staff of recent examples of their occurrence, with specifics.

5. There are strong tendencies toward the status quo; deviate from the norm and create time and space to brainstorm and encourage new ideas when people are out of their normal routine and environment.

6. People tend to conform; have systems in place to inform everyone that the majority of staff are complying with the new policy.

7. Stating an intention publicly increases its likelihood of occurrence; publicly share goals or have staff individually indicate that they intend to participate in a change.

In general, we can create choice architecture to encourage certain decisions over others while still fostering autonomy and purpose and providing rewards in the form of praise, feedback, and additional information. An appropriate choice architecture for routine tasks might allow individuals to complete the task in their own way while acknowledging that it is mundane but necessary.

When we fully examine the concepts described in this chapter, we begin to see how they link together. Behavioral economics taught us how individuals process information through automatic and reflective systems. We applied that theory to the different heuristics and examined how inherent biases influence individuals' evaluation of a situation. Utilizing both, we are able to employ "nudges" through choice architecture to influence someone's behavior. We understand from the work of psychologists and behavioral economists that it is important to allow for individual preferences, emotions, and motivations. A nudge is most realized when it is habit forming, although it requires building trust, supporting basic needs, and positive interaction to thrive.

We have touched on the fact that individuals are influenced by the interactions they have with others, and that the level of interactions scale non-linearly with the size of the organization they inhabit. Armed with the tools from this chapter, we can shift focus and more readily examine these theories as they interact within an organization. Scaling up, we will explore how the behavior of systems as a whole is influenced through the choices and actions of the individuals within.

Chapter 5

Complex Adaptive Systems

The task of accurately describing the system of a typical healthcare delivery organization is a daunting one. As individuals come together to form a larger organization or system, we observe that the quantity and complexity of their interactions increase. Additionally, the aggregated product or output of the system as a whole is more than could be expected from the sum of their independent activities. This observation is certainly true within healthcare delivery, as individual doctors and nurses rely on the collective resources, skills, and knowledge of their entire organization. We also know that the physical environment of a hospital or clinic, its resources, geographic location, and surrounding community play crucial roles in the level of care available to patients. These healthcare delivery systems have their own unique cultures, organizational structures, and even social networks influencing how individuals interact, cooperate, and collaborate.

In Geoffrey West's book *Scale*, social networks described in a typical company or city involve a hierarchy of groups that increase in size and decrease in strength as they move outward from the individual (e.g., family group, friend group, acquaintances, larger surroundings, etc.). Within these groups exist "nodes," individuals networked to each other through a series of social links; "hubs" arise out of those nodes and represent individuals with the most connections. These concepts, too, are applicable to a healthcare delivery setting within the various departments, divisions, and physical locations of larger healthcare systems. The relevant model of a healthcare delivery system is one that reflects the complexity of interplay between several key areas:

- individual interaction
- physical environment
- social and cultural dynamics
- impact of internal and external forces related to budgets, regulations, and guidelines
- knowledge and understanding of diseases and their treatment

The field of complexity science encompasses numerous theories and frameworks exploring how systems with multiple components interact with each other. These systems may involve biologic processes (e.g., the human brain), ecological systems (e.g., climates), or, as discussed previously, social systems such as cities, companies, and organizations. In addition to the notion that characteristics of a collective system are different (and often greater) than those of the individual components, some complex systems are also able to adapt and evolve in response to changing conditions. This category of systems, commonly referred to as Complex Adaptive Symptoms (CAS), has received considerable interest in recent years because of its applicability to many national and international challenges. The framework of the CAS appeals to those in a variety of disciplines due to its acknowledgement of both system dynamics and the importance of individual member behavior.

Specifically stated, a CAS is an open, dynamic network of semiautonomous individuals who are interdependent and connected in multiple non-linear ways.

COMPLEX ADAPTIVE SYSTEM

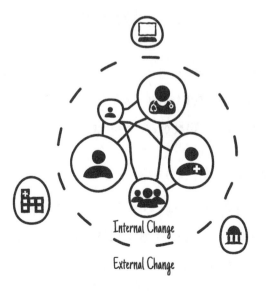

Internal Change

External Change

The behavior of a CAS is not defined by the individual components (i.e., people) but by the interactions between the members and others *within* the system as well as their interactions with *external* forces. On the surface that sounds technical, but if we explore the definition a little further it's a reasonable description of almost any healthcare delivery system. As mentioned previously, a healthcare delivery system such as a hospital has multiple departments (emergency services, critical

COMPLEX ADAPTIVE HEALTH CARE SYSTEM

A NETWORK THAT IS OPEN, DYNAMIC, FLEXIBLE, ADAPTIVE AND COMPLEX.

COMPLEX DUE TO
Numerous interconnected, semi-autonomous, competing and collaborating members.

ADAPTIVE DUE TO
Capability of learning from prior experiences
Flexibility to change its members connecting patterns to fit better with its surrounding environment

care services, surgical services, pharmacy, administration, etc.) where dozens or even hundreds of individuals have a variety of duties and responsibilities. Almost all of these are in some way connected to the duties and responsibilities of others throughout multiple departments. Obviously, members in this system interact with each other, although each unique set of circumstances may require different interactions with different members and across different departments or hierarchies.

To more fully understand what we mean, consider the actions and interactions of staff when a single patient walks into the emergency department. Within minutes (hopefully), the patient encounters multiple staff and triggers the creation of a paper or electronic trail that will document and track the health encounter from beginning to end. Once evaluated, the patient might require hospital admittance for an overnight stay, where additional services are provided, such as lab tests, imaging, or even surgical procedures. After treatment and sufficient recovery, the patient is ready for discharge, which requires additional services, staff, resources, and coordination. Over the course of that healthcare encounter, the number of individuals who interact—directly or indirectly—as a result of this one visit is considerable: physicians, nurses, lab techs, administrators, coders, and potentially pharmacists, physical therapists, patient advocates, social workers, and others.

While the individuals who take part in providing care are semiautonomous in completing their roles along the patient's journey, staff are clearly interdependent and likely to have multiple interactions with each other of varying intensity and duration. However, since no two healthcare delivery systems are identical in their staffing, facilities, or resources, not to mention their geographic area, vicinity to other services, culture, and patient populations, they are unlikely to produce the exact same set of interactions. From the view of a CAS, healthcare delivery organizations are unique in their member diversity and culture, member interactions, surrounding environment, and previous history.[22]

A CAS has the ability to adapt and evolve in response to changes in its environment (internal and external) by learning from prior experiences.[23,24] As such, the capability of the organization to adapt to internal and external changes depends on individuals' characteristics as well as local organizational structures and environment. This is a key factor for why a CAS provides an accurate framework for healthcare delivery organizations. The CAS recognizes that organizations are

CHALLENGES ADDRESSED
BY CAS PRINCIPLES

- HOW CAN I MANAGE THE PROBLEMS OF UNCERTAINTY, VARIABILITY AND VARIABLE INTERDEPENDENCE?

- HOW CAN I IDENTIFY AND SELECT A MEANINGFUL CHANGE?

- HOW CAN I EVALUATE THE SUCCESS AND THE IMPACT OF MY PROPOSED INTERVENTION OR CHANGE?

not static—they face constant change both internally and externally. Internally they may face changes in staff, the physical environment, or resource allocation. Externally they might grapple with new regulations, important research findings, or variations in case-mix or the health of patients. The individual members' capabilities, as well as attitude and aptitude for alteration, will determine how skillfully and efficiently the system as a whole can adjust and acclimate.

When viewed in the light of CAS theory, it becomes clear that the success of any implemented change relies on its ability to function and thrive within a system of unique individuals. Additionally, we can immediately see that evoking a desired change does not so much require a change to the "system" but to the decisions and interactions of the individuals who make up the system. (Consider what we have previously learned about how choice architectures can help influence those individual decisions and interactions.) Further, CAS theory also promotes the idea that individual departments or divisions are not separate or independent components. Instead, change within part of the system will likely have repercussions throughout the entire system, to a varying degree. Therefore, when implementing a change, it is crucial to consider and monitor its impact on the system as a whole.

We can see that the concepts inherent in CAS theory apply to healthcare delivery systems by allowing their complex nature while still acknowledging the autonomy of the individuals and considering an ever-changing landscape of regulations, health policy, and practice guidelines. When combined with the lessons from behavioral economics, heuristics, and choice architecture, we can begin to picture how to evoke desired change in a physical and social environment. However, we must also understand the role played by variability—not just in the uniqueness of individuals, but also from multiple sources at multiple levels throughout the system.

Chapter 6

Variability in Care Delivery

Sources of Variation

Earlier we discussed how a healthcare delivery organization is a complex adaptive system. Each one consists of unique individuals interacting and collaborating in a myriad of different ways. We also explored how biases in automatic cognitive processing provide insight into creating a choice architecture effective at encouraging certain decisions and behaviors. In this chapter, we acknowledge that the process of delivering care is inherently variable and that the variability stems from multiple sources.

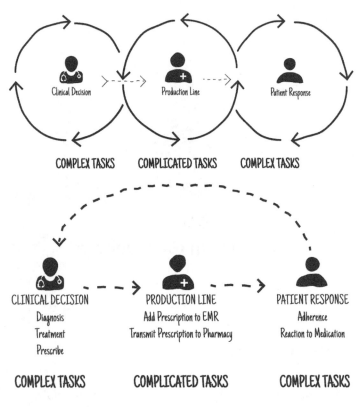

Specifically, when we consider the delivery of a typical healthcare service, we can identify three main sources of variation in clinical care.[25]

The first of these is variation in clinical decision. Often, making a clinical decision (e.g., a diagnosis, a recommendation for treatment and follow-up, etc.) involves multiple providers and is a function of accumulated clinical knowledge, experience, and accepted or emerging practices. Let's consider an example to illustrate.

When a patient presents with chest pain at the emergency department, that patient may see multiple providers who attempt to identify the source of discomfort through a variety of methods (performing an exam, asking questions about medical history, employing diagnostic tests). The provider attending to this patient leverages their own specific skills to determine the sequence and extent of each activity. It is likely that the provider will use their reflective cognitive process to consider possible diagnoses and to estimate the risk of certain outcomes based on specific patient characteristics such as age, gender, and medical history. These considerations embody a unique and personal interpretation of current or emerging care practice guidelines and result in the provider deciding on the best course of action for this patient. Other providers may interpret symptoms and risk factors slightly differently or consider certain practice guidelines to be more or less applicable to the situation. Experience also plays a pivotal role in the variation between health professionals, which can ultimately result in a difference in care a patient might experience from that provider forward.

Once they make a clinical decision, the second source of variation involves the process of translating the clinical decision into patient care. The speed and competency with which care delivery applies will be a function of several important factors. The providers' skill and experience, resources available at the facility, and any process or system in place to expedite care or ensure quality are all examples of such factors. Should the patient presenting chest pain be admitted, there will be variation in the timing of that event based on several elements both clinical and administrative. If, on the other hand, the patient is discharged, there will be a need to coordinate the procedure, relay the discharge instructions (including special directions or prescription information), and possibly provide prescription filling services. For each of these tasks, there exists a multitude of ways to navigate a completion. Staffing levels, existing standardized processes or procedures, and even an individual's unique characteristics can have significant impact on a patient's experience and the efficiency of their visit. As we examine what goes into procedures like intake and discharge, it becomes clear where significant variability can occur and, in some cases, become the deciding factor in an operation's efficacy.

The final source of variation is the patient's response to the healthcare services. Both the patient's clinical characteristics (age, disease burden, level of cognitive impairment or frailty, etc.) and their inherent attitudes and opinions have impact on their clinical response and ability to implement treatment. In addition, patient behavior regarding diet, exercise, lifestyle, and other factors contributes to the effectiveness of a treatment and improving (or at least stabilizing) the patient's health. Although many of these factors are outside the control of a provider or medical facility, it becomes possible to influence patient behavior by drawing on the lessons we have learned in previous chapters.

Understanding these sources of variation and how they can affect care delivery is crucial when attempting to implement effective and sustainable care solutions.

Five Factors Framework

We acknowledge that we are not the first to develop a model for effective and sustainable implementation of healthcare solutions. On the contrary, our success builds upon a foundation laid by others who have struggled to identify and describe the key elements of successful interventions. In a 2013 paper, Chaudoir, Dugan, and Barr[26] summarize previous implementation frameworks and note that many suggest multilevel factors influence the likelihood of success for a given intervention. They categorize these factors into a hierarchy from a macro- to a micro-level:

At the macro level is an external sociocultural structure-level factor that includes aspects of the setting or community surrounding the organization. Examples include the physical environment (including geographic location, urban versus rural, etc.), the political and social climate, public policies, the current economic strength, and local infrastructures. These factors tend to influence the patient population an implementation might target or the administrators a team needs to secure demand with in order to get their strategy off the ground. Most of these factors will not be readily alterable and instead require thoughtful tactics to leverage their unique position in a plan to maximize intended effect.

On a deeper level, beneath the external sociocultural structure, is a factor inherent to the organization itself. Comprised of all its aspects, the organizational-level factor is usually where implementation of a particular innovation or solution occurs. It includes things like organizational culture, the leadership's ability to guide the organization, and the general morale of staff. These factors may be more within the control of an implementation team to alter. Not necessarily consisting of permanent aspects such as geographic location or the wider politics of the area, these factors are endemic and unique to each organization and can be pushed or influenced by the right individuals working in concert. While not always easy to manipulate, these factors are important to a team attempting implementation as any new change might alter these conditions.

Within the organizational-level factor exists the provider-level factor, reflecting the characteristics of the clinician or group involved in implementing the solution. As stated previously, skills and capabilities vary across individuals, as do attitudes and opinions. Some may have more faith in practice guidelines, techniques, or evidence-based practices, which influences their ability to effect change in care delivery within their immediate circle of influence.

At the most micro level are the innovation-level factor and patient-level factor. Not all innovations are as cost efficient, user friendly, or efficient as others. The quality of the idea itself is a core factor in the success of an implementation. Additionally, numerous patient characteristics can influence the success of an intervention. Sometimes an idea can struggle to gain traction against negative elements such as education level, health-related beliefs, motivation, behavior, and innate attitude toward medical care and health-related innovation.

It is understandable when the authors go on to note that any combination of these factors can influence the success of an implementation. Fidelity, level of adoption, penetration of the solution, cost, and sustainability are alterable at any level of factor category. By understanding the five factors framework, one is able to identify and develop measures to evaluate the factors and define how they might interact or influence an implementation outcome. With that tool, we complete our ensemble and can finally discuss the system that brings it all together, Agile Implementation.

Part III
SPECIFYING THE MODEL

Chapter 7

The Agile Implementation Model

F rom the experiences of the Healthy Aging Brain Center, the Critical Care Recovery Center, and the Central Line Associated Bloodstream Infection reduction project, we accumulated the knowledge and understanding of key elements in the implementation process that increased the likelihood of a successful and sustainable implementation of evidence-based healthcare solutions. Our examination of relevant theories and frameworks illuminated what we observed firsthand regarding how a healthcare delivery system functioned and the roles played by the unique members and providers who delivered care. Across the theories explored in the previous chapters, the common message is that healthcare delivery systems are complex, adaptive, and sociotechnical.

Successfully implementing changes requires an approach that attends to:

1. variation that is both temporal (across process steps) and hierarchical (across levels of the system and care-delivery process);
2. the human element and human-to-human or human-to-technology interfaces; and
3. the way organizations function in and adapt to the broader sociocultural, legal-political, and organizational-regulatory environments.

When conceived of in August 2011, the Indiana University Center for Health Innovation & Implementation Science (IU-CHIIS) aimed to understand and utilize implementation science tools to facilitate clinical change and tackle the issue of increasing knowledge head-on. The multidisciplinary team convened as part of the IU-CHIIS was able to draw on a wealth of experience and knowledge to leverage and unite the concepts, theories, and frameworks described in the previous chapters. That expertise coalesced into a comprehensive and cohesive model for identifying and implementing innovative care solutions. The final product is a result of considerable effort, led by a network of dedicated individuals. These colleagues supported the exchange of information and ideas across partner systems and facilitated the development of training and mentoring programs for providers, researchers, and healthcare delivery system administrators.

In this chapter, we present the details of the Agile Implementation (AI) model, which involves eight steps rooted in the theoretical frameworks described in previous chapters. Each step allows for the uniqueness of each healthcare delivery system (from CAS theory) and recognizes that variation in clinical decisions, translations into patient care, and patient responses (from sources of variation theory) will influence the impact of a solution. The AI model leverages aspects of behavioral economics and the sociocultural and multilevel factors described in the Five Factors Framework to guide interactions and evaluations. Agile Implementation encourages individuals to act in ways that enable the success and sustainability of the selected solution.

The eight steps are as follows:

Step 1: Identify Opportunities
Step 2: Identify Evidence-Based (EB) Healthcare Services
Step 3: Develop Evaluation and Termination Plans
Step 4: Assemble a Team to Develop a Minimally Viable Service
Step 5: Perform Implementation Sprints
Step 6: Monitor Implementation Performance
Step 7: Monitor Whole System Performance
Step 8: Develop a Minimally Standardized Operating Procedure

The eight steps of the AI model are facilitated by a trained AI agent. These agents can be internal to the organization (e.g., a

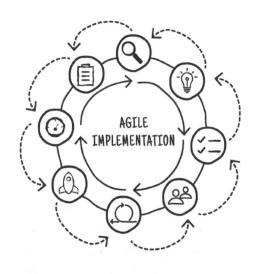

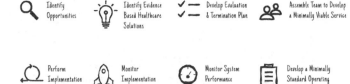

	Identify Opportunities		Identify Evidence Based Healthcare Solutions		Develop Evaluation & Termination Plan		Assemble Team to Develop a Minimally Viable Service
	Perform Implementation Sprints		Monitor Implementation Performance		Monitor System Performance		Develop a Minimally Standard Operating Procedure

clinician or administrator) or external (consultant). Each agent knows how to identify an appropriate EB solution and is able to facilitate changes at both the organizational level (zooming out) and the individual level (zooming in). Often the AI agent benefits from receiving formal training in one or more aspects of the model, such as the underlying theories and frameworks, conflict resolution, and deeper implementation strategy. These trained agents are experts in leveraging the AI system in a variety of circumstances within their own organization and the new ones they encounter. Each becomes capable of transforming a workforce, through the AI methodology, into an efficient implementation team and spreading those lessons through each new individual influenced.

We describe the details of the individual steps below, including the role of the AI agent in each step and examples of how these activities look in an actual implementation.

Step 1: <u>Identify Opportunities</u>. The first step of the process is to identify and confirm the presence of an opportunity. Too often we try to establish change before sufficient 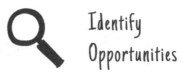 demand for that change is established. While everyone welcomes the idea of improved care as a concept, restrictions related to finances, regulations, and staffing can derail efforts before they even begin. This kind of false start can doom not only the immediate intervention but may also reduce enthusiasm for future efforts if staff perceive attempted implementations as "half-baked." Therefore, to identify opportunities, the AI agent proactively works with leadership and clinical providers to understand the needs and goals of the organization. A gap in care quality indicates potential for an opportunity, but not necessarily its viability as a potential project. The AI agent must also establish high demand for the solution within the organization, identified when executive leadership and frontline clinical providers volunteer to invest the time, personnel, and financial resources necessary to pursue the opportunity.

To illustrate, recall that prior to the formation of the HABC, leadership at Eskenazi performed a cost analysis to determine the financial viability of the solution, and the CEO gave the ultimate go-ahead. Similarly, when exploring the ICU survivor opportunity, key stakeholders of Eskenazi were cognizant of similar trends with this type of care in the larger healthcare environment. After analysis, they recognized it as a potentially marketable attribute of the facility. To garner support and establish sufficient demand within the organization, leadership and key stakeholders must be able to envision how the solution will benefit the organization's underlying objectives and long-term financial health, in addition to improving patient care.

Step 2: <u>Identify Evidence-Based Healthcare Services</u>. After

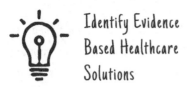

Identify Evidence Based Healthcare Solutions

identifying an opportunity and establishing demand within the organization, the AI agent conducts a systematic search to identify EB healthcare services. These services must address the selected opportunity and promote the quadruple aim (high-quality, accessible, cost-efficient, and patient-centered care) for the patient, family, and providers. It is critical to understand that the AI model requires the use of proven solutions, as this stands as a major departure from other implementation strategies. You may be familiar with other methodologies that encourage solutions born from anecdotes, personal experiences, or brainstorming sessions. The only solutions used in the AI model are those that have been sufficiently tested and demonstrated to be effective empirically. Most often, identifying potential EB solutions involves searching published literature and practice guidelines or examining the recommendations of industry specialists or policy makers. When searching and evaluating potential EB solutions, we recommend employing a critical appraisal like the grading process used by the US Preventive Services Task Force to determine the quality and strength of the supporting evidence.

To improve dementia care, the HABC team was able to draw upon two randomized clinical trials that demonstrated the effectiveness of the collaborative care model, while the CLABSI reduction project utilized known and established clinical care guidelines published by the CDC. For each of these projects, the proposed solutions were evidence supported and highly regarded organizations (like the CDC). These types of solutions have immediate credibility with staff and can foster buy-in and confidence in the proposed intervention.

Step 3: *Develop Evaluation and Termination Plans*. At this point in the process, the team has identified both the opportunity and the EB

✔ — Develop Evaluation
✔ — & Termination Plan

solution. The following steps reflect the activities necessary for applying and tracking a solution through the local environment in a way that acknowledges and considers the unique delivery system and its members. In Step 3, the AI agent works with organizational leadership to develop an evaluation protocol and selects the measures appropriate to the organization, service type, implementation goals, scheduled milestones, and indicators of success. Step 3 requires that the AI agent fully understand the implications of implementing the proposed change, from the smallest micro-level to the highest macro-level, including potential implications for the surrounding community and related organizations. Establishing reliable and valid measures requires an understanding of the Five Factors Framework, the sources of variation theories, and their application to the complex interconnected nature of the delivery system. These measures need to provide timely feedback to frontline providers, have the capacity to signal and identify unintended consequences or benefits, and still allow leadership to evaluate broader impacts to the financial well-being of the organization. Ultimately, the evaluation plan must specify the criteria for de-implementing the planned EB healthcare service as early as possible. An essential part of Step 3 is identifying the criteria for determining the implementation a failure and establishing both the method of de-implementation and who will lead it.

During the HABC implementation, the team examined both clinical and cost data to understand revenue generated by the new program and the cost savings associated with preventing acute-care utilization events. To evaluate the CCRC implementation, the team tracked quarterly data on antidepressant use and cognitive function, along with system-wide readmissions, ED use, and a variety of cost measures. Those involved in the CLABSI reduction project understood the likelihood of a spillover effect in other areas of patient harm events and proactively tracked rates of multiple infections and other types of harm events.

Step 4: _Assemble a Team to Develop a Minimally Viable_

Assemble Team to Develop a Minimally Viable Service

Service. Even if the EB solution was developed and tested within a setting and for a population similar to that of the intended implementation, the uniqueness of the local environment requires a tailored and adjusted variant. The AI agent bases the solution on the characteristics and make-up of the organization, its members, and its patient population. Therefore, in Step 4 the AI agent works with leadership to build a local interdisciplinary and diverse implementation team to convert the selected EB service(s) into a *minimally viable service*. This team localizes both the content and delivery process to ease implementation. These are the "minimum" specifications, meaning that when the team finalizes the process, it needs to incorporate these specific aspects to maintain the fidelity of the EB solution. Therefore, the interdisciplinary team must understand the EB solution well enough to pinpoint the essential features and attributes to retain locally. Developing the minimally viable service is a collaborative process, and the team understands that the service will be iteratively revised and refined in subsequent steps.

For the HABC, this manifested as a list of seven specifications for Alzheimer's care within the Eskenazi Health including education, periodic needs assessment, medication management, and care coordination. To arrive at these specifications, the team utilized the expertise of diverse staff to oversee the program. The interdisciplinary team consisted of experts in Alzheimer's care including a primary care physician, three geriatricians, a nurse, a social worker, two neuropsychologists, a social psychologist, a clinic administrator, and a representative from the local Alzheimer's Association. The CCRC project saw its team built from several experts in pulmonary/critical care and geriatric medicine. As discussed in the study, these members were chosen for their use of collaborative care models in Alzheimer's disease, depression, and other geriatric syndromes.

Step 5: __Perform Implementation Sprints__. After the initial

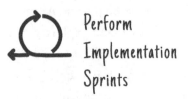

version of the minimally viable service is developed, Step 5 begins to incorporate the solution into the care delivery process. This step evaluates the solution's performance and identifies aspects that need further adjustment or alteration. Implementation truly begins at this stage. An AI agent facilitates self-contained "sprint" cycles, which are short, intense cycles of implementation designed to test the components of a plan by enacting them at a local level. After a sprint, staff provide feedback regarding their experience and discuss potential adjustments they feel would make the process more effective and sustainable. A team makes appropriate modifications before the next sprint, and this process continues iteratively until all are satisfied the component is at its most effective for the local environment and intended use. Changes to the specifications of the solution may be small or large. Full participation is critical for the sprints, and the staff must feel comfortable sharing their experiences and feedback regarding process improvement. The AI agent plays a crucial role in this context because he or she will need to weigh the needs expressed by frontline providers with the restrictions and parameters set in place by the larger organization regarding budget and timeline.

During the development of the services provided by the HABC, we hired additional staff when sprints revealed that nurses and social workers were often unavailable to provide adequate care coordination because they were too busy administering neuropsychological testing to new patients. The team implementing the CCRC responded to high rates of no-shows by adding a process for direct referrals and phone calls to better acclimate new patients to the program.

Step 6: _Monitor Implementation Performance_. During the implementation period, a need for continuous feedback exists regarding the success or failure of the implementation. Therefore, Monitor Implementation Performance

during this step the AI agent and the implementation team develop feedback loops to monitor the fidelity and performance of the selected service. Reflection on what the team is learning through the process often focuses around gauging impact and acknowledging any conflict or tension. Identifying emerging problems leads to prioritizing their solutions to adjust the implementation process and sprints accordingly.

During the CLABSI intervention, we held multiple meetings with units that struggled with performance on metrics of incidence rate and catheter days. Teams reviewed data from clinical dashboards and, with the help of specialized staff, identified areas for improvement and developed specific plans for those improvements.

Step 7: _Monitor Whole System Performance_. In addition to the continuous monitoring of the performance of the service itself, the AI agent and implementation Monitor System Performance

team must also monitor impact of the implemented service on the overall quality and financial performance of the entire organization. It is essential to detect any unintended or adverse consequences of implementing the service, but also to identify any emergent opportunities of additional benefit.

The HABC team evaluated impacts to revenues and costs during the program. Similarly, the CCRC team set up regular performance feedback loops to determine effects on the system as a whole and to monitor clinical outcomes and processes. The CLABSI reduction implementation team tracked rates of other infections and patient harms to detect potential spillover effects.

Step 8: <u>Develop a Minimally Standardized Operating Procedure</u>. If the imple-

Develop a Minimally Standard Operating Procedure

mentation met internal demands and goals, then the AI agent and implementation team develop a *minimally standardized operating procedure* manual. The team updates the manual on a regular basis and helps spread the successful services across other departments within the same organization or across other organizations.

After the first year of the HABC, procedures stabilized and the team created a minimally standardized operating procedure. With this in hand, the HABC program could be evaluated against the manual to ensure long-term implementation.

Healthcare 2.0

The methodology described in this book represents the culmination of decades of work and study by countless dedicated individuals. From a personal standpoint, I view the Agile Implementation model as a critical tool for revamping the healthcare delivery system into one that consistently provides high-quality, high-value, and accessible care for all patients (Healthcare 2.0). Accomplishing this goal requires a tightly connected network of passionate, resilient, skilled change agents who can leverage the concepts and theories presented above. Through sustained effort, we can transform healthcare delivery organizations into responsive and learning systems, and can inspire and nurture a level of care I had only imagined was possible those many years ago when I was first being trained as a physician.

To assist committed change agents, we have developed specialized tool kits to help learn and employ the Agile Implementation Model steps in real-world settings and situations. These tool kits include guides to help confirm demand within your organization, develop a plan for the evaluation and monitoring of your intervention, and construct the minimally viable service, among other things. The Appendix includes several of these items, and for those who are interested in further developing their proficiency with the Agile Implementation model, we offer training certifications through the Center for Health Innovation & Implementation Science at Indiana University (this information is also in the Appendix).

Thank you for joining me on this journey; this work is personal to me and reflects much of my time, effort, and passion. I hope you will find it to be transformative for you and your patients, and I am excited for all I believe we can achieve together.

About the Authors

Malaz Boustani, MD, MPH, is the Founding Director of the Sandra Eskenazi Center for Brain Care Innovation Center and the Founder and Chief Innovation and Implementation Officer of the Indiana University Center for Health Innovation and Implementation Science. The center's mission is to generate innovations to improve patient care as it tackles systemic healthcare costs. To this end, he leads a diverse and interdisciplinary team of scientists, clinicians, and engineers to develop and implement innovations that improve brain health, brain care quality, and patients and their families' brain care experience. He is also a Research Scientist for the Regenstrief Institute and a Professor of Medicine at the Indiana University School of Medicine. Dr. Boustani lives in Indianapolis with his wife Mary and has two children, Katreen and Zayn.

Joze Azar, MD, is the Chief Quality and Safety Officer at the IU Health Academic Health Center as well as the co-founder and Chief Engagement Officer at the Center for Health Innovation and Implementation Science. He is also a practicing Hematologist/Oncologist at the IU Health Simon Cancer Center. He graduated Medical School from the American University of Beirut in Lebanon, completed his Residency in Internal Medicine and Fellowship in Hematology/Oncology at Indiana University School of Medicine in Indianapolis, IN. He lives in Indianapolis with his wife Karen and two children, Christopher and Nicole.

Craig A. Solid, PhD, is the Owner and Principal of Solid Research Group, LLC in St. Paul, MN. He has worked in healthcare research and quality for twenty years, focusing on issues related to data, measurement, and value. He lives in St. Paul with his wife Emily and their three children, Vieva, Emmett, and Kipp.

Appendix I
Suggested Reading

Books

The Innovator's DNA by Jeff Dyer, Hal Gregersen, Clay
    Christensen
Nudge by Richard H. Thaler, Cass R. Sunstein
Drive by Daniel H. Pink
The 4 Disciplines of Execution by Chris McChesney Sean
    Covey, Jim Huling
Thinking Fast & Slow by Daniel Kahneman
The Undoing Project by Michael Lewis

Articles

Azar J, Kelley K, Dunscomb J, et al. Using the agile implementation model to reduce central line-associated bloodstream infections. Am J Infect Control. Jan 2019;47(1):33-37.

Azar J, Adams N, Boustani M. The Indiana University Center for Healthcare Innovation and Implementation Science: Bridging healthcare research and delivery to build a learning healthcare system. Z Evid Fortbild Qual Gesundhwes. 2015;109(2):138-143.

Boustani MA, Munger S, Gulati R, Vogel M, Beck RA, Callahan CM. Selecting a change and evaluating its impact on the performance of a complex adaptive health care delivery system. Clin Interv Aging. May 25 2010;5:141-148.

Boustani M, van der Marck MA, Adams N, Azar JM, Holden RJ, Vollmar HC, Wang S, Williams C, Alder C, Suarez S, Khan B, Zarzaur B, Fowler NF, Overley A, Solid CA, and Gatmaitan A. Developing the Agile Implementation Playbook for Integrating Evidence-Based Health Care Services Into Clinical Practice. Acad Med 2019;94:556-561.

Khan BA, Lasiter S, Boustani MA. CE: critical care recovery center: an innovative collaborative care model for ICU survivors. Am J Nurs. Mar 2015;115(3):24-31.

Appendix II

Confirm Demand Guide

Insert score from 1 to 100 for each demand domain. Add domain scores to get the total score. Divide total score by 6 to get the adjusted score

Score

Executive support

Service line/administrative engagement

Clinician engagement

Strength of supporting evidence

Impact to the quadruple aim

Potential to scale up

Total

Grade Scale

90-100	= A
80-89	= B
70-79	= C
60-69	= D
<60	= F

Projects Demand Score should be B or greater to be considered for selection.

Appendix III

Implementation Guide

Problem Statement

_____

Solutions Name

_____

Target State Metrics

Metric	Baseline	Target

Create Implementation Plan & Implement

O Introduce the Innovation Project, review the Project Narrative, and present selected solution

Person Responsible	Start Date	Completion Target	Completion Date	Current State and Next Steps

O Share Project Team Member Expectations

Person Responsible	Start Date	Completion Target	Completion Date	Current State and Next

O Share meeting frequency and locations

Person Responsible	Start Date	Completion Target	Completion Date	Current State and Next Steps

O Share Project Timeline

Person Responsible	Start Date	Completion Target	Completion Date	Current State and Next Steps

O Share Communication Plan

Person Responsible	Start Date	Completion Target	Completion Date	Current State and Next Steps

Identify Resources needed for Implementation

Identify Resources Needed

Create Implementation Plan & Implement

O Identify steps to implement goal

Person Responsible	Start Date	Completion Target	Completion Date	Current State and Next Steps

O Identify Lead Person for each step that is accountable and responsible to implement or delegate

Person Responsible	Start Date	Completion Target	Completion Date	Current State and Next

O Identify a timeline for each step

Person Responsible	Start Date	Completion Target	Completion Date	Current State and Next Steps

O Begin creation of the SOP as project progresses

Person Responsible	Start Date	Completion Target	Completion Date	Current State and Next Steps

Create Evaluation Plan

O Identify process to regularly collect project metric data, as defined on the Project Narrative

Person Responsible	Start Date	Completion Target	Completion Date	Current State and Next Steps

O Identify interim goals and benchmarks

Person Responsible	Start Date	Completion Target	Completion Date	Current State and Next Steps

O Identify metrics and process to monitor the health system impact

Person Responsible	Start Date	Completion Target	Completion Date	Current State and Next Steps

O Develop reporting timeline

Person Responsible	Start Date	Completion Target	Completion Date	Current State and Next Steps

O Develop reporting format

Person Responsible	Start Date	Completion Target	Completion Date	Current State and Next Steps

Refer frequently to Project Timeline

O Utilize Project Timeline to stay on track

Person Responsible	Start Date	Completion Target	Completion Date	Current State and Next Steps

O Revisit timeline routinely

Person Responsible	Start Date	Completion Target	Completion Date	Current State and Next Steps

Refer Frequently to Communication Plan

O Use Communication Plan to keep stakeholders informed and educated

Person Responsible	Start Date	Completion Target	Completion Date	Current State and Next Steps

O Revisit Communication Plan routinely

Person Responsible	Start Date	Completion Target	Completion Date	Current State and Next Steps

O *Insert detailed tasks required to address*

Person Responsible	Start Date	Completion Target	Completion Date	Current State and Next Steps

Finalize the Standard Operating Procedures, Policies, Protocols

O For all new processes, develop Standard Operating Procedures, Polices and/or Protocols

Person Responsible	Start Date	Completion Target	Completion Date	Current State and Next Steps

O Share SOP to other areas to Scale and Spread

Person Responsible	Start Date	Completion Target	Completion Date	Current State and Next Steps

O *Insert detailed tasks required to address*

Person Responsible	Start Date	Completion Target	Completion Date	Current State and Next Steps

Additional Tasks

O *Insert detailed tasks required to address*

Person Responsible	Start Date	Completion Target	Completion Date	Current State and Next Steps

Appendix IV

Evaluation Guide

This form is meant to guide you through the evaluation planning process. Review Evaluation & Termination Criteria and revise as needed to incorporate elements from the selected solution keeping in mind the following elements:

Overall Evaluation

Are there available controls (i.e. other sites within the system, other clinics within the site, etc.)?

Design will be a comparison of implementation sites with control sites; regression analysis to compare change over time across the two types of sites?

Yes ⭕
No ⭕

Yes ⭕
No ⭕

Do you have Historical Data?

Yes ⭕ Can do interrupted time series, regression testing, traditional pre-post analysis, etc. based on whether or not repeated measurements are available?

Yes ⭕
No ⭕

No ⭕ Can only look at change post-implementation and will need good process measures to show change due to implementation?

Yes ⭕
No ⭕

Monitoring

Run-charts and Control Charts are used to monitor processes and outcomes?

The charts can be processed throughout the entirety of the implementation period?

Yes O

No O

Yes O

No O

Outcome-Process Linking

Regression analysis to look at process measures effect on outcomes

O Can look at variables individually or together in one analysis

O Can identify which processes work best

Qualitative Comparative Analysis (QCA)

O Different type of analysis using mathematical algorithms

O Recently being used more in implementation research

O Used to identify which combination of components from a multifactorial intervention have the most impact on the outcome

Appendix V

Monitoring Guide

Monitor the impact of the selected solution on the outcomes of the entire system. Check assumptions regarding your evaluation criteria/plan and the intended value proposition

Continuous Review of Defined Measures

O Review primary and secondary outcome measures on pre-determined intervals (weekly, monthly, quarterly, etc.) based on anticipated project length

O Continuous review of defined measures

O Determine if measures are acceptable based on thresholds

Examples

Best case scenario:

Quality ▲   Cost ▼

Worst case scenario:

Quality ▼   Cost ▲

Mixed scenario 1:

Quality ▼   Cost ▼

Mixed scenario 2:

Quality ▲   Cost ▲

Appendix VI

MINDSPACE GUIDE

MESSENGER
We are heavily influenced
by who delivers information

SALIENCE
We are drawn to information
perceived to be novel and relevant

INCENTIVES
We are very loss adverse

PRIMING
We are impacted subconsciously
by environmental cues

NORMS
We are strongly impacted
by our perception of what
others are doing

AFFECT
We go with our gut feelings;
our first, emotional reaction

DEFAULTS
We go with the flow and tend not
to change preset options given

COMMITMENTS
We seek to be consistent with
our public promises

EGO
We want to feel good
about ourselves

Minimally Viable Solutions Guide

Insert score from 1 to 100 for each demand domain. Add domain scores to get Total Score Divide Total Score by 6 to get the Adjusted Score

Score

Meets Quadruple Aim

Cost-Effective

Time Constraints

Resource Commitment

Executive Level Support

Operations Level Support

Total

Grade Scale
90-100 = A
80-89   = B   Score should be B or greater to
70-79   = C   be considered for selection.
60-69   = D
<60   = F

Appendix VIII

LEAN	PDSA	AI	What Differentiates Agile Implementation	
✖	✖	✓	Manages interface between internal and external environments	★
✖	✖	✓	Confirms demand from end-user	★
✓	✖	✓	Identifies evidence based-solutions	
✖	✖	✓	Determines the criteria and timeline to stop a failed solution	★
✓	✖	✓	Localizes the content, processes, and outcomes	
✓	✓	✓	Develops a timely and actionable feedback loop	
✖	✓	✓	Monitors impact of the solution on the system	
✖	✖	✓	Monitors emergent behaviors	★
✖	✖	✓	Maintains a minimal standard operating procedure	★

Graduate Certificate

 Are you ready to become a Certified Change Agent?

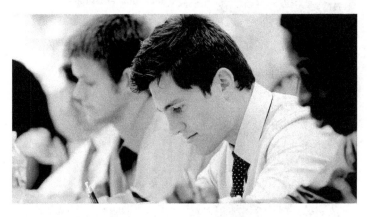

Health Innovation and Implementation Science Graduate Program

Offered by the Indiana University School of Medicine

www.hii.iu.edu/change

Build a foundation with core courses. Apply and refine your knowledge through practicums. Build your network while exchanging ideas with your cohort and faculty in person at the on-campus weekend residencies.

References

1. Balas EA, Boren SA. Managing Clinical Knowledge for Health Care Improvement. *Yearb Med Inform.* 2000(1):65-70.

2. Grant J, Green L, Mason B. Basic research and health: a reassessment of the scientific basis for the support of biomedical science. *Res Eval.* 2003;12:217-224.

3. Ebell MH, Sokol R, Lee A, Simons C, Early J. How good is the evidence to support primary care practice? *Evid Based Med.* Jun 2017;22(3):88-92.

4. *Best Care at Lower Cost: The Path to Continuously Learning Health Care in America.* Wasington DC: National Academy of Sciences; 2013.

5. Alzheimer's Association. 2018 Alzheimer's Disease Facts and Figures [internet]. 2018; https://www.alz.

org/media/HomeOffice/Facts%20and%20Figures/ facts-and-figures.pdf. Accessed 2019 Apr 22.

6. Bremer P, Cabrera E, Leino-Kilpi H, et al. Informal dementia care: Consequences for caregivers' health and health care use in 8 European countries. *Health Policy.* Nov 2015;119(11):1459-1471.

7. Valimaki TH, Martikainen JA, Hongisto K, Vaatainen S, Sintonen H, Koivisto AM. Impact of Alzheimer's disease on the family caregiver's long-term quality of life: results from an ALSOVA follow-up study. *Qual Life Res.* Mar 2016;25(3):687-697.

8. Callahan CM, Boustani MA, Unverzagt FW, et al. Effectiveness of collaborative care for older adults with Alzheimer disease in primary care: a randomized controlled trial. *JAMA.* May 10 2006;295(18):2148-2157.

9. Vickrey BG, Mittman BS, Connor KI, et al. The effect of a disease management intervention on quality and outcomes of dementia care: a randomized, controlled trial. *Ann Intern Med.* Nov 21 2006;145(10):713-726.

10. National Quality Forum. Endorsement Summary: pulmonary and critical care measures. 2012; www. qualityforum.org/Projects/Pulmonary_Endorsement_ Maintenance.aspx

11. Desai SV, Law TJ, Needham DM. Long-term complications of critical care. *Crit Care Med.* Feb 2011;39(2):371-379.

12. Cuthbertson BH, Roughton S, Jenkinson D, Maclennan G, Vale L. Quality of life in the five years after intensive care: a cohort study. *Crit Care.* 2010;14(1):R6.

13. Khan BA, Lasiter S, Boustani MA. CE: critical care recovery center: an innovative collaborative care model for ICU survivors. *Am J Nurs.* Mar 2015;115(3):24-31; quiz 34, 46.

14. Vital signs: central line-associated blood stream infections--United States, 2001, 2008, and 2009. *MMWR Morb Mortal Wkly Rep.* Mar 4 2011;60(8):243-248.

15. Rupp ME, Majorant D. Prevention of Vascular Catheter-Related Bloodstream Infections. *Infect Dis Clin North Am.* Dec 2016;30(4):853-868.

16. Furuya EY, Dick AW, Herzig CT, Pogorzelska-Maziarz M, Larson EL, Stone PW. Central Line-Associated Bloodstream Infection Reduction and Bundle Compliance in Intensive Care Units: A National Study. *Infect Control Hosp Epidemiol.* Jul 2016;37(7):805-810.

17. Azar J, Kelley K, Dunscomb J, et al. Using the agile implementation model to reduce central line-associated bloodstream infections. *Am J Infect Control.* Jan 2019;47(1):33-37.

18. Kahneman D. Maps of Bounded Rationality: Psychology for Behavioral Economics. *American Economic Review.* 2003;93(5):1449-1475.

19. Thaler RH, Sustein CR. *Nudge: Improving Decisions about Health, Wealth, and Happiness.* Yale University Press; 2008.

20. Chaiken S, Trope Y. *Dual-process Theories in Social Psychology.* Guilford Press; 1999.

21. Kahneman D. *Thinking, Fast and Slow.* Farrar, Straus and Giroux; 2011.

22. Boustani MA, Munger S, Gulati R, Vogel M, Beck RA, Callahan CM. Selecting a change and evaluating its impact on the performance of a complex adaptive health care delivery system. *Clin Interv Aging.* May 25 2010;5:141-148.

23. Anderson RA, Crabtree BF, Steele DJ, McDaniel RR, Jr. Case study research: the view from complexity science. *Qual Health Res.* May 2005;15(5):669-685.

24. Hagedorn H, Hogan M, Smith JL, et al. Lessons learned about implementing research evidence into clinical practice. Experiences from VA QUERI. *J Gen Intern Med.* Feb 2006;21 Suppl 2:S21-24.

25. Azar J, Adams N, Boustani M. The Indiana University Center for Healthcare Innovation and Implementation Science: Bridging healthcare research and delivery to build a learning healthcare system. *Z Evid Fortbild Qual Gesundhwes.* 2015;109(2):138-143.

26. Chaudoir SR, Dugan AG, Barr CH. Measuring factors affecting implementation of health innovations: a systematic review of structural, organizational, provider, patient, and innovation level measures. *Implement Sci.* Feb 17 2013;8:22.

CPSIA information can be obtained
at www.ICGtesting.com
Printed in the USA
BVHW041312090919
557933BV00001B/1/P